Contents

Who would give me my best reference?

Who would give me my worst reference?

The Super You Project

INTRODUCTION

New Joiners' Brief

Understanding fitness and what it means to you personally can be quite a profound learning process. Most people these days gauge their fitness on how they look, but fitness goes a lot deeper than this.

I am going to be completely honest with you. My main reasons for improving and maintaining my fitness and keeping my waistline trim are:

1. To be able to spend time with my family taking walks, climbing trees, etc with few functional limitations (which is tough, considering my injury profile – but I do my best).

2. To feel good in social environments with friends and family. There is nothing better than praise about how good you look – just take a glance at Instagram. (There is a fine line, though, between wanting to look your best and plain old narcissism.)

3. To be in shape for family holidays and have confidence in my body as I walk onto a beach.

So, how do I achieve maximum outcome with little time commitment? Through smart training and creating a process that serves my goals, that's how. This same approach has helped dads all over the world to achieve their fitness and fat loss goals.

Generally, we are used to being told that it only takes a small amount of time to get fit and stay fit. Just look at the best-selling fitness books of all time – they are all based around achieving good outcomes in minimal time. What they tend to leave out, though, is the amount of mind management it takes to build into your life the strategies that enable fat loss and fitness success to happen. To succeed with these programmes, you must be mentally resilient and believe strongly in *why* it is important for you to succeed in your fitness and fat loss goals. Once this is established and the power to create change (or to maintain it, for those who are on their journey already) outweighs the power to stay as you are, then you have taken a positive step towards attaining your goals.

It must be made clear: sacrifice is a definite part of fitness. I use the word 'sacrifice', but I quite enjoy the discipline and self-control involved. Whatever we call it, you already know that this is what it takes to succeed at anything in life – buying a house, sending your kids to university, etc. What are we sacrificing? Time, mostly. Who wouldn't want to spend more time with their family, with their partner or watching *Game of Thrones*? One of the main things we look at when adopting the approach described here is what activities we are spending the 24 hours in our day on. What I am highlighting here is your choices – your behaviour. This could be limiting you and preventing you from maximising the effects of your fitness and fat loss journey.

What I have learned (and what science supports with regard to building a psychological environment that will lead to a positive fitness state) is that success is a case of *marginal gains*. You have to take a holistic approach and make sure you have all the bases covered. That's why it's essential to have a system that is easy to understand and follow.

Think of the approach as a map. Maps are only useful if you plan your route and also any detours. During my explanation of the approach, I provide you with the map you need to guide you to your desired destination: loving what you see in the mirror without the BS shakes and pills.

Effort is rewarded with results

The dads who have followed this approach have seen rewards for their efforts. This is no quick 'get fit in thirty days' programme or '6-minute abs' routine. No, sir. This is total, brutal honesty. This is the dads' no-BS approach to fitness and fat loss.

There are eleven steps in this process. These provide you with the information that will enable you to make the best decisions and maximise effectiveness in your fitness journey.

Fat loss and fitness, or fitness and fat loss, regardless of your priorities and goals, in this blueprint you will find a route that will guide you – if you put it into practice. Will it guarantee you results?

Results are what I specialise in.

I've worked in the military for seventeen years (twelve years as a Petty Officer Physical Trainer and five years as an Exercise Rehabilitation Specialist). I know what makes people tick, and I know the excuses that most people make and how these get in the way of their progress. It takes effort to make changes, but the effort does not go without reward.

The blueprint to becoming the unstoppable dad your kids brag about

Think of this approach as the foundation of what is required to get you on track in your fitness journey. I run the Super You Dads' Online Fitness Community, which has dads breaking down barriers and hitting excuses out of the park. The dads who join have a lifetime membership and go through the steps I outline systematically to ensure they are fully loaded and capable of succeeding. They are challenged every month with physical tasks and goals. They are encouraged to be consistent and are supported by all the other dads in the community (the key ingredient for most fitness success).

But we are not here to discuss the online community right now. We are here to help you prepare for the start of your lifelong fitness journey. What follows is how we are going to guarantee the success you deserve.

Step 1: Start with one thing

During this step, you will learn that it doesn't take much to get started and how just changing *one thing* at a time leads to greater success. This step also breaks down goals for the future. I will discuss ways to avoid overwhelm and break through the barriers of excuses.

We keep everything plain and simple. No BS. You will discover how some dads have used this approach to change their lives and how others have made mistakes that you need to avoid.

Step 2: Swap steps for MEPs

The world now revolves around technology. The little devices in everyone's pockets can be either our friends or our foes. What I mean by this is that too many of us spend far too much time scrolling through social media, watching meaningless content and allowing these devices to take over our lives.

What if we could use this technology to our own advantage? What if we used it to help us become more in tune with our health and fitness? Wearable technology has been one of the biggest trends of the last few years. I use a specific wearable with all my clients these days, especially within the online community. The reason is that it enables us to measure effort objectively and gauge whether we deserve the results or not.

Myzone tracks effort and gamifies fitness to encourage better engagement, and this step explains how. I will tell you the story of when Frank the MEP (Myzone Effort Points) Tank met Mac Attack during one of the monthly challenges I set, how they both told me they didn't have much time to work out – and how, despite this, they managed to do 73 hours of exercise each in one month.

Step 3: Motion is the lotion

'Motion is the lotion' is one of the key principles within the community. Movement triggers a chain reaction that helps people get on track with not just their fitness but their lives (powerful stuff). It's simple: getting off your arse to move more is the perfect start to building a healthier lifestyle. This is where the principle of 'start with *one thing*' is most influential. Keeping it basic and mastering the fundamentals is critical for long-term engagement in fitness. Too often, I see dads overcomplicate their workouts and end up failing to stick to anything.

During this step, we highlight the power of walking daily. We look at how to find time in your super-busy schedule. Every dad is busy, but never too busy to get a session in the bag. We also look at how keeping on your feet as much as possible will help you torch calories more efficiently throughout the day. You will also learn how to boost your results by increasing intensity, and the importance of having a leg day in your exercise programme to minimise injuries.

Step 4: Better mood, better food

By Step 4, you will have started to be consistent with your exercise and are likely to notice that your mood has elevated. When we are in a better state of mind, we tend to make better choices – in theory, the feel-good chemicals released during exercise will elevate our mood. When making decisions around food, you may therefore find your behaviour starts to drive success in your fat loss and fitness journey.

There are a few things I regularly point out to the dads I work with. A lot of them come to me with pre-existing beliefs and barriers to success that I have to put to bed. Some of the main (and most frustrating) beliefs are that if the food is healthy, they can eat as much of it as they like; that counting calories is old science; and that if they are training for half an hour a day, they can pile their plates high. I always remind dads that calories count even if you don't count them.

In this step, I will give insight into food-preparation hacks and how to leave the leftovers before they go straight to your waistline. As the old saying goes: a moment on the lips, a lifetime on the hips.

A few other subjects we will cover include why shopping on an empty stomach is not the best idea, and how efforts made during the week can easily be devastated by beer and junk food at the weekend.

Step 5: Binger vs consistency ninja

By Step 5, you will have recognised whether you are a binger or a ninja. If you are a binger, the time to do something about it is right now.

The binger will work hard in the gym, prep food like a boss, and cycle to work every day for a week... And will think that this is enough for the month.

The ninja, on the other hand, is cut from a different cloth. The ninja is fully aware that the tortoise wins the race and that taking his time and relying on principles like 'start with one thing' and 'consistency builds momentum' are what will ensure a lifelong healthy lifestyle. The ninja never gets distracted.

Step 6: Treat yourself like you'd treat your nan

Something that happens to us parents all too often is that we forget to take care of ourselves. The way I see it, how can you expect to feel like the best dad if you're not feeling like the best you?

I'm all for prioritising family, but if your family is to benefit from you being the best version of yourself, that has to involve paying some attention to your own health and well-being. Many dads tell me after just a few weeks how awesome they feel and how positive their family's response has been towards their transformation. Treating yourself as well as you would treat your nan if you took her on holiday puts a different spin on how you handle your own health.

Finding a balance between movement and munch and understanding the techniques needed to ensure your mental and physical health have to be at the forefront of your thinking, rather than just being something in the background. This is covered during this step.

Step 7: The fat loss gremlins

There are certain factors involved in creating a successful fat loss strategy that are commonly missed – things that go under the radar and that you might not have considered.

During this step, you will learn that running is not as good a strategy for fat loss as some people claim, that running could in fact be killing your lean gains, and that there are better ways to become a leaner version of yourself. You will discover that by overcomplicating things, you are less likely to succeed – the pressure of thinking about too much at once may cause your plans to stall. (This brings us back to our main theme: start with *one thing*.)

There is also a particular issue I want to highlight, but it can be personal, so I need to tread carefully. Hopefully, by this stage, we will have built a strong enough bond for me to raise this issue: some dads find that their partner has been sabotaging their results. An unsupportive partner can crucify progress by making life difficult and guilt-tripping you when you need to get a session done.

Lastly, we cover the fact that patience (which seems to be an unfashionable concept) is what will help you succeed when the going gets tough. Remember, fitness isn't a destination; the end goals can change, so we have to be patient during the times when we see little progress and evaluate and change the game if necessary.

Step 8: Plateau isn't a place in Greece – nor is it a place in fat loss

You've now hit the dreaded plateau. Only, I don't believe there is such a thing. We now need to dial in and get serious. There are a few things we need to consider once we get deeper into our fitness and fat loss progress.

Dads often forget to adjust their total daily energy expenditure. This could have you eating up to 500 calories more per day than you need. If you have a significant amount of weight to lose and have lost 10–15 kg in eight weeks (I see this all the time, by the way), your brain will panic. It will start to think this is the new normal and may drain you of the motivation to move. This is the brain fulfilling its most primitive function: preserving life at all costs. Although logically you know that you are eventually going to maintain a healthy weight you are happy with, your brain may not understand this.

Being more aware of sitting time and becoming geekier in tracking your steps will give you objective feedback on how much you're moving. This is also the time to become aware once again of eating the leftovers, or that biscuit you didn't track in the staff room, or that handful of the kids' sweets at the cinema. It's time to review these things and be honest with yourself.

This step will also include our first discussion of sleep. It can be a touchy subject, but there is a lot of evidence that points to the benefits of a good night's sleep and the effects on stress levels.

We will finish this step with a story about how excessive cardio has the opposite effect to the one you're aiming for.

Step 9: Obsessed with accountability

It is amazing how some people make throwaway comments to others, such as, 'You're obsessed with that fitness craic' while sitting on their arse eating a tub of Ben and Jerry's and watching some programme like *The Only Way Is Essex* on the box.

To become better and change anything in life, there *has* to be an element of obsession. This sparks motivation. Yes, obsession can be detrimental to your health if you are obsessed with the wrong things (drugs, alcohol, etc). But for me, a healthy obsession with exercise gets a big thumbs up.

What has been interesting to observe in the Super You Community is the dads' obsession with accountability. How they win bragging rights by being consistent in their fitness journeys. Quite remarkable, really.

Step 10: Sex, sleep and rock 'n' roll

Sex has a hugely positive impact on mental health and reduces stress levels. It also has the ability to increase testosterone levels, which helps build muscle. That said, when dads experience weight gain, sex can be neglected and can become another contributor to the negative mindset that makes it difficult to get started on the path of taking positive action.

Although we touched on the issue of sleep a few steps back, here I'll talk about how sleep hygiene is crucial for recovery – how you can gain better results with a good sleeping routine, even if it is disturbed. I was in denial for so long when it came to sleep. My little girl, even now, is up at least once in the night for a toilet break or calls out because Doris the dragon has fallen out of bed. It's soul-destroying when you have a baby who sleeps all day and is up all night. On those days when you're sleep-deprived, the last thing you want to do is get your kit on and beast a workout. Here, once again, we'll see the power of *just one thing*.

Having a healthy sex life alongside getting a decent night's kip are not the only hacks for staying healthy, mentally and physically. Scheduling date nights more often can also play a role in increasing our motivation – I'm speaking from experience on this one.

Step 11: Do epic shit to raise money

Imagine going your whole life and barely scratching the surface of what your body is capable of doing. Most of the dads I come across tell me either that they are past it and that their best days are behind them, or that they don't believe in themselves, point blank. They don't make excuses, they just don't feel confident that they can make a positive change to their lives.

In the Super You Community, after we have encouraged the dads to start with one thing, they get the wind in their sails. They start believing that the negative messages they were telling themselves were just BS and obstacles they were putting in the way of becoming the super versions of themselves. Many of them then challenge themselves further. They start doing epic shit. They start dedicating their blood, sweat and tears to a bigger purpose. A cause. They start doing their bit for charities and raising awareness for research projects that can help fight cancer. This is what I call 'next-level shit', where you put yourself in uncomfortable situations, all for a greater cause.

STEP 1
Start With One Thing

What you are about to read will explain one of the most important aspects of making changes to your health. Too often, I see clients fail because they become overwhelmed by the structure they have built around themselves.

Start with *one thing*. Then see where that takes you.

Hell, yeah! I can somersault over a 6-foot box

Starting with *one thing* was something I learned through my own experience with injury in my military career.

In 2006, I passed a two-day selection course to become a Royal Navy physical trainer. I have to say, it was the most brutal two days of my life physically (not mentally; the worst for that was another course, the Joint Service Exercise Rehabilitation Instructors' Course – for another time, maybe). By the end of Day 1, we had done so much exercise I had burned between 10,000 and 12,000 calories. From repeated back-to-back fitness testing to climbing a 30-foot rope, the two days were epic. The selection test taught me the true range of what a human body can manage, physically.

That said, once I passed the aptitude test and was selected for the next course, I had an encounter with injury. I was playing a game that only northern Spartans of the M62 (for my overseas readers, the M62 is a motorway running across the north of England) would recognise. That game is Rugby

League. High-impact and fast-paced, the game takes no prisoners and has never been kind to my body. I went down like a sack of spuds on the field and was rushed to hospital. They took an X-ray of my knee but couldn't see much. Weeks later, I got back to semi-fitness and was still hopeful of getting on to the physical trainer course. I played in another Rugby League game (I know what you are thinking now: dickhead), and the knee buckled. I was, yet again, in a heap on the floor.

I finally had an MRI scan (which is able to see ligament damage). It confirmed that the anterior cruciate ligament had fully ruptured and that the ligament behind it didn't look too pretty either. Surgery it was, then.

I was broken. I'd been through exercise rehabilitation before and knew it was tough to get back to even half the fitness standard you'd been at before. I began to grow anxious about my future. Wondering whether the injury was going to end my career, my fate with regard to the physical trainer's course seemed sealed.

I was drinking heavily for the first few weeks after surgery and had written everything off – until I bumped into a lad who was undergoing rehabilitation in the same unit. He'd had a below-knee amputation and wanted to get back to running. He was adamant.

I felt guilty. Here was a guy who had a prosthetic leg, and I was moaning because I'd had a ligament reconstruction. I stopped thinking so far into the future and started with just *one thing*. The one thing I started with was fifty press-ups a day. I managed that for a week. Then I started with fifty pull-ups a day. Next, I did upper body circuits and began my knee rehab.

Before I knew it, I felt awesome. Within four months, things were looking a lot brighter. Yes, I had constant pain, which I never discussed with anyone in the medical team. Yes, the knee ballooned every time I ran. But I started with just *one thing* and took it one day at a time. By the end of the physical trainer's course, I was able to somersault over a 6-foot box.

All this was achieved by starting with just one thing.

JOSH'S MISTAKE

Josh wanted to take his fitness and fat loss seriously, as his wife had just given birth and he wanted to look good for their first family holiday. He started at the gym. He biked to work. He meal-prepped every night. He went back to playing football. He started training at the weekend before the family were up.

He set himself all these goals. Then, after five nights with no sleep because of the new baby, he drove to work. He negotiated with himself that he would drive to work and spent an extra hour being restless in bed. He said to himself that he would go straight to the gym after work. Then he had the day from hell. Nothing went right, and time disappeared into the usual black holes. He eventually got home, went straight to the fridge, opened a can of beer, went to the cupboard, opened the crisps and sat on the sofa. 'Netflix and chill – I deserve this,' he told himself.

Because Josh had goal-stacked himself, he ended up negotiating with himself and compromising everything at once. He decided that he would start again the next week, giving himself credit because he had managed three weeks of consistent training. While those three weeks were a remarkable achievement, and I do applaud him for this, they would mean nothing if for the rest of the month he did zero exercise, zero portion control and zero tracking of his movements throughout the day.

He would find it hard to get back into the swing of things and would convince himself he was past all this 'fitness game', being a dad – and besides, the dad bod is cool. (It is absolutely not cool.)

When people first start their fitness journeys, they roll out a massive list of goals.

They start off with the best intentions, but then, as life throws a spanner in the works (which it always does), the first thing they compromise on is their fitness. They tie everything related to fitness – food, gym, etc – together. What I tell them to do is to pick just one thing and start with that.

MATTHEW STARTED WITH JUST ONE THING

Of all the conversations I've had with the dads I have worked with, one in particular comes to mind. Matthew never made the mistakes that dads like Josh always make. He started with just one thing.

Matthew is a 32-year-old, hard-working guy with two kids and a wife. He lives in the north of England. When he was younger, he carried some weight around his midriff, but was never severely overweight – certainly not in his early twenties. He played Rugby League, training twice a week and playing at the weekend. He loved his booze. In fact, he still loves his booze.

Towards his late twenties, the weight started to creep on more and more. He got married and had two kids. Time for any type of exercise or sport drained from his routine. Although his job was still active, the stress of work, being a dad and providing for his family began to open the seams, and he developed a dependence on food and alcohol to self-manage the chaos inside his head. Before he knew it, he was 109 kg and felt like rubbish.

When I decide to set up the Super You Community, I had dads like Matthew in mind: dads who just need that little bit of encouragement to review what's not working in their lives and what we can do about it. When Matthew contacted me in October 2018, he was quite sheepish and a little embarrassed. (Most dads are; this is another reason why it takes them a long time to ask for help.) He told me he didn't feel 100%. He wanted to start getting in shape for his boys, and he felt something in his lifestyle needed to change. He wanted to feel fit and get back into the shirts that had been sitting in his wardrobe since his early twenties.

I asked him what he needed to do to make this happen. I asked him how he could get in shape. He was confused at first. 'I thought you were going to tell me,' he said.

'I don't need to. Everyone knows the basics, and that's what I always work with,' I replied. 'Do you mean cut down on the booze and junk and get my arse to the gym?' he asked. 'Well, even more simple than that to start with. I don't want you to feel overwhelmed in a few weeks,' I explained.

Matthew started with my recommended daily power walk. He committed to doing the minimum of a power walk once a day at least five days a week. Within four weeks, he had lost 7 kg. His surprise that simply sticking to one thing would change the number on the scales was satisfying to witness.

This is the power of just one thing. It means having something (fitness-related) in your routine that you never negotiate on. It has to be something simple.

Depression and just one thing

When I started the Super You Dads' Online Fitness Community, I had no idea how honest the men would be within that type of group setting. As I write this, one dad sticks out in my mind. He came to the group coaching system like a beast unleashed. He started with the power walking, but before long he was cranking it up with some awesome home workouts. He lost 10 kg and was really building momentum.

We had discussed the fact he had struggled with depression for quite some time and that he was aiming to transition, with guidance from his doctor, to a minimal dose of antidepressants. I could tell he was worried about not hitting it hard like he had been for the past few months and that he was scared of slipping back into his old ways. We reviewed what the whole process is based upon – starting with just one thing. We acknowledged that sometimes we may have to go back to basics just to keep things ticking over while other issues take priority.

What was important about this situation for me as a coach was that he felt supported by the community and was reassured that making the decision to stick with just one thing would pay off in the end.

Coaches' corner

Starting with just one thing is that first step that almost every client I have ever worked with has previously missed out. They want a big long list of audacious goals to start with and don't recognise that just *one thing* is better than what they are already doing on a weeknight (which is probably watching Netflix and scratching their ballsack).

Once you can get your head in the game with something small and be consistent with it, it's time to move on to more things to challenge yourself.

Swap Steps For MEPs

I'd like to take the time during this step to give you some insight into how technology is taking the dads in my online community's fitness to the next step.

Space is ace

Let me make this crystal clear: I love technology and how it is leading us into the future. I love movies like *Total Recall* and *Interstellar*. I try to imagine what it would feel like to travel in space, how the body would feel and the impact being completely weightless could have on the digestive system – or any bodily system, for that matter. With the technology we have made on Earth so far, the possibility of true space travel is becoming more likely than ever before.

My sci-fi interest doesn't stop with outer space travel. Can you can remember the old movie *Inner Space* with Dennis Quaid back in the 1980s? The movie where Quaid is zapped by a device that shrinks him, and he ends up navigating around the human body for a short while? This still gets my juices flowing, and we are discovering more and more about the human mind and body all the time.

This is why I am so fascinated with the current trend in the fitness industry. Fitness-related wearables have been the biggest, fastest-growing trend of the past five years because they provide people with live and recorded feedback on their fitness performance over various disciplines of sport and physical activity. Pedometers have long been used as a measurement tool; some say that Leonardo Da Vinci conceived of the idea, and that the first pedometer was used in the 1700s. It wasn't until 1965, though, when the Japanese realised the correlation between steps taken and calories burned, that the devices became popular. Today, the wearable fitness technology is so advanced that you can wear a watch that can all but tell you how many farts you've done.

On a serious note, though, in healthcare settings, fitness wearables have started to be considered tools that could have a positive impact on society's biggest health risks, such as lack of physical activity.

Gamification

Anything that can be measured can usually be used as black and white data to gauge progress – certainly in the fitness world. I've known big businesses all over the UK reward their workers with monthly prizes using step counters on various gadgets (eg smartphones).

Steps seem to be the easiest, most popular and least expensive way to measure physical activity. In addition to the specific wearables available for this, there are countless free smartphone apps that measure motion and track every step you take. Measuring steps and making a game out of the data collected is a clever way to take advantage of the competitive nature of the human mind – if you think you are not competitive, you're lying to yourself. Think of a league scenario: whoever gets the most steps wins the league – get it? It may sound simple, but the fact of the matter is: simple works. Simple gets results – in this case, a smaller waistline. What else is out there that can measure fitness progress? How else can we gamify fitness?

There are a whole range of different trackers available these days that measure a variety of data from the human body. The favourites tend to be those that evaluate heart rate and effort, and give feedback on how many calories have been burned during a fitness session. One device I have discovered in the last few years is called Myzone, which I mentioned earlier. If there were a gold standard for wearables that make fitness fun, this one would, without doubt, be top of the list.

Discovering Myzone

I came across the Myzone fitness tracker around three years ago. At the time, I was delivering a military-style bootcamp for an exclusive female-only residential camp. I met a lady there who kept bringing out her phone after the sessions, and I became more and more intrigued. (I wondered if she was Instagramming while in instruction – naughty!) I eventually went over to her after an epic beasting (standard during camps like this) and asked her what she was looking at on her phone (hoping she wouldn't say something embarrassing). Was it business? Was she expecting an important phone call from home? She said: 'It's my stats on Myzone.' 'What's that?' I replied.

She went on to explain how the whole process worked and how motivating she found it. I picked up on the key word 'motivating' and asked her to explain how the device achieved this. Her explanation of the heart rate-based measurement system and the points rewarded for certain effort zones had me captivated straight away. I loved the idea of being rewarded for your effort and also having kudos amongst friends in the Myzone community. At the time, I couldn't figure out where it would fit with the clients I was currently working with. (I was working in exercise rehabilitation for the British Armed Forces.) I knew, though, that it was something special and something I could use for myself and for my clients in the future.

'Mac Attack' vs 'Frank the MEP Tank'

Find a problem, then solve it.

That is what my business mentor told me. I have a burning desire to help the nation – hell, help the world – become more active, more often. I've had this desire for as long as I can remember. Looking around at the fitness industry, there is a clear map of those who have had the greatest impact on the largest number of people. Any physical trainer who has had huge success in helping people fulfil their fitness goals has had a significant online presence and talked about fat loss, not just fitness (although fat loss, as a rule, is a side effect of good fitness). One of the most successful physical trainers with an online presence is Joe Wicks, author of several cookery and fitness books.

Like Joe, I have also written books. They are for children, and the intention –
which I achieved – was to sell them to schools, to inspire kids to do more
exercise and become aware of how important functional movements are in
the lifelong journey of fitness. They are cool, even if I do say myself. But the
books alone weren't enough to get the message fully into households. I had to
think of something that grabbed parents' attention, too.

Some years later, and after a few meetings with various mentors, the idea of
building an online fitness community was first raised. I envisaged a fitness
community that was incredibly simple yet highly effective; one that would
excite the audience and also excite me. It's important to enjoy what you do,
after all.

First, I needed to define the specific audience. I thought about it and
discussed it with an awesome copywriter friend, Mike Samuels. I came up
with the demographic of dads over thirty. I knew these were the people I
could help the most and relate to the best. Their pain points are lack of time,
lack of motivation, and always putting the family first. The consequence is
that they sacrifice their own health and fitness.

Once I knew who I wanted to work with and where I could make the most
impact, the next thing to consider was how I could clearly stand out from the
many misleading and sometimes unethical fitness concepts out there. Just
being honest with the dads was a good start, but I also knew exactly how I
could get these dads off their backsides and straight into their gym kits. You
guessed it: Myzone. Myzone is what the dads I work with spend time getting
to grips with and the thing that sparks the motivation of the Super You
Community. It creates challenge.

When I first started to write the workouts for the community and think about
how I could guide the dads with good solid information about how to get the
most out of their training, never in a million years did I think they would take
the challenges so seriously that they would take days off work to win a
challenge. These are dads who own their own businesses, who had told me
they didn't have 30 minutes a day to train. It's crazy to think that the dads
who were at first struggling to get off the sofa and get to the fridge to open

another can were now out in the great outdoors at every opportunity to earn Myzone Effort Points (MEPs) – the measurement system used to reward participants.

In the first few months, there was one dad who was always holding the top spot. At first, it was a little disheartening for some guys. Although the dads found value in the live feedback and tracking their progress along with all the other support they were getting (food intake guidance, mind management, etc), there was still a feeling that when I set the new challenges each month, there was only going to be one winner. This dad even earned the name 'Frank the MEP Tank'. I found this highly amusing.

Then, out of nowhere, the tide turned. An old Navy friend approached me through social media and asked what Super You was all about and whether he could join. Once I explained the ins and outs, he was fully on board (pun intended). Within a week of his first challenge, he had made Frank the MEP Tank's efforts look mediocre (well, maybe that's a bit harsh). The buzz this created in the group was outstanding. The other dads started to believe that, with the right mindset, it was possible to make that much effort in their fitness journey, that Frank the MEP Tank was not an abnormality.

That challenge created a great sense of competitiveness and also comradeship. The new dad used to box for England and had earned the title 'Mac Attack', and he certainly still had that discipline lurking below the surface.

Coaches' corner

While some fundamentals remain true when it comes to achieving long-lasting results, the world is moving fast with regard to fitness. Wearable technology is proving to be a valuable data source that can point scientists in the right direction when considering external factors that motivate people.

Giving people something that they can have in front of them providing live feedback on their performance elevates the effort made during sessions; like Mac Attack vs Frank the MEP Tank – I'm sure both checked the MEPs (if you're still confused, check out www.myzone.org) during their sessions to see how many more points they needed to win.

From a fitness point of view, wearables are becoming the norm and are a way of building communities within a workout environment. Myzone has 'gamified' exercise by rewarding users; it uses a points system and league tables to reward those who make more effort to condition themselves.

Motion Is The Lotion

I'm often criticised within the fitness industry for simplifying the fact that if people moved more often, the problems that society are plagued with would be halved. Hear me out on this one. If people actually got off their backsides and walked to the shops, by the time they got there they'd feel better after the rubbish day they'd had at work. Because of their elevated mood, they'd be less inclined to sabotage the 'feeling good' moment by eating the 18-inch double cheese pizza and may go for the 12-inch instead (small steps).

What am I saying here? Movement influences mood, so if I can get people moving more often, that's a great start, even if that's just a walk (remember: start with *one thing*).

Born to walk

Moving our bodies – getting around under our own steam – is what we are born to do. Things were different back when our ancestors had to scavenge for food and protect their communities; when there were no common places to take cover and the wild was a lot wilder than it is today (although there are some scary sights on Instagram). We had chemicals in our bodies that were driving our responses to the types of threats we faced.

- We had adrenaline to activate our 'you'd best fight or run, or you're going to die' response.

- We had endorphins that were released into our system as pain relief after running from danger.

- We had dopamine to give us that boost of achievement after we had caught our food or managed to escape the beast that was chasing us.

- We had oxytocin that drove us to build relationships with others, build communities, and make life easier – two heads are better than one, right?

These chemicals haven't gone anywhere. They still form the basis of most of our responses and decisions in today's world. But our environment *has* changed. We no longer chase food – it is delivered to our front doors. 'Danger' is worrying whether someone liked your last post or whether that picture saved to the cloud and, if so, whether your partner will see it. Yikes. Relationships are based on swiping right or left, rather than on the need to find a suitable cavemate. And, in the environment we have built for ourselves, moving our bodies is hardly necessary.

We have forgotten that Mother Nature built us for endurance, and that we love success. The chemicals in our bodies will allow us to walk for miles and miles if we want to – ever heard of the 'Man versus Horse' race in Wales?[1]

In our hunter–gatherer days, people would probably have jumped at the chance to hunt, purely because they were addicted to the runner's high. The 'runner's high' is the release of endorphins, our body's natural pain relief. The hunters would have got a double hit once they'd caught their food, too, because dopamine, the hormone released when we are successful in something, is highly addictive. This 'achievement hormone' is the one that most successful people are addicted to.

As you can see, we are made to exercise.

Walking is more than losing extra weight

In 2017, I got the devastating news that my dad was dying. He had cancer.

As you can imagine, this had a profound effect on my life. Watching this mountain of a man go from 106 kg to less than 70 kg had a huge impact on my mental health. The self-reflection I engaged in during the period immediately after my dad's passing had me turning myself inside out and questioning everything. My emotions were so overwhelming that every day I had to battle the urge to hit the bottle. Alcoholism runs deep in my family, and unfortunately it is something I must counteract on a regular basis.

At the time I couldn't think straight, so developing a programme for myself was not top of my list of priorities. I knew I had to do something, though. I knew I had to get out of the slump. When I was younger, running would have been the easiest thing to do, but having had so many injuries over the years, running triggers a lot of symptoms for me. I thought, what do I usually start my clients with? I often start them (depending of the injury, of course) with walking – again, this is going back to basics and starting with just one thing. At first, I thought, let's see if I can manage an every-other-day thing.

I enjoyed it. I downloaded the Runkeeper app on my iPhone so I could track my pace, and after 30 minutes I was dripping wet from holding a pace of 14-minute miles. Then it became a daily thing. I found that, the more I walked, the more stuff I figured out, and I began to accept that my dad had gone. Day by day, it became less painful, and the urge to drink was subsiding as I built momentum and stayed consistent with my daily walk. I had created a peaceful place within my mind. After walking for 30 minutes each day, I would feel at peace with what had happened instead of wanting to go out and destroy myself finding the bottom of a bottle. What was happening here?

My theory is that, rather than giving in to the urge to drink my way through the pain, I was replacing it with something that was cheaper and healthier, had no negative consequences, and was more positive for me, my family, my friends and, most importantly, my little girl.

Once I began to observe the mental health benefits of walking for myself, I started to preach its virtues to my friends and family. I told them how it made me feel and how it had contributed to my weight loss, which was pretty drastic – in the time since my dad died, I have lost 16 kg using a holistic approach, including daily walking.

At work, I got a small group of blokes together, and we would walk in the mornings before work – chatting about manly stuff, obviously. At weekends, I would invite my best friend, who I'd played rugby with throughout most of my life, to go for a power walk along the beach. We both watched the weight fall off our waists and found ourselves walking into Saturday mornings with our families, feeling like a million dollars.

I am now a firm believer that walking is the king of mind management and building bonds with friends and family. This is exactly why it is the starting and fundamental exercise of the Super You Community.

It's simple. It's free. It costs you calories, not money. Absolute winner.

Stay NEAT and keep on your feet

My grandad was always a fit old soul. Even though he would knock back a whisky or two on a rare occasion (who am I trying to kid? It wasn't rare, he liked a whisky most evenings), he still managed to reach his eighties. During the winter, I would notice he would put on a few extra pounds, and I always thought he must be letting his age catch up with him. But then every summer he would 'lean down' to his fighting weight – my grandad loved to spin a yarn about his boxing days, when he was serving his queen and country.

It wasn't until I saw him one day in his garden that I put two and two together. He worked all through the spring and summer in his garden. He did it every day, from sunrise to sunset. He didn't stop there, either. He did the rounds of the entire street he lived on and kept all the old folks' gardens shipshape.

What my grandad was doing here didn't involve making any drastic changes to his diet or setting aside time for specific exercise. By providing a service and keeping on his feet, he was moving more. It may seem strange to you when I talk about gardening in the context of weight loss, but activities like this can be considered Non-Exercise Activity Thermogenesis (NEAT).

I'll explain. First, let's define a calorie:

> 'A calorie is just a measure of a unit of energy; technically speaking, it's the energy required to heat 1 litre of water by 1 degree

centigrade.'[2]

It's a fact that when you are moving more, you are burning more calories. Simple. The intensity with which you burn those calories is another story altogether.

With this in mind, every time the Super You dads ask me about losing weight, I always recommend they up their NEAT levels by doing things like resisting the craving to just sit on the sofa when they get home; by being more active and doing things around the house, or anywhere else.

Are we sitting ourselves to death?

Dr Kelly Starrett's book *Deskbound: Standing Up for the Sitting World*[3] has radically changed the way I look at the act of sitting. Although I have always delivered a strong message about moving purposefully, this book has increased my knowledge and understanding of the ever-growing problem of inactivity.

Within the book, there are three recommendations in particular that Starrett has got absolutely right and which could help solve the general problems that come with too much inactivity (maintaining the same posture for too long – sitting or standing):

1. Reduce optional sitting in your life

2. If you must sit, move every 30 minutes for 2 minutes

3. Perform 10–15 minutes of daily maintenance on your body (eg yoga poses)

What does this mean?

Obviously, the following won't apply to everyone. If this is nothing like your typical day, I apologise in advance. However, this is a typical sedentary day for many people. Picture yourself waking up in the morning. After you have been to the toilet (2–5 minutes of sitting), you go downstairs to sit and eat breakfast (10–15 minutes of sitting), you drive to work (30 minutes of sitting), you get to work and sit in the coffee room with colleagues (10 minutes of sitting). Then, you sit at work for around 10 hours (depending on what job you do). You drive home (30 minutes of sitting), get in, and sit down in front of the TV to have dinner. You stay there until you go to bed. Sound familiar?

We need to reduce the proportion of our days we spend sitting. How? Picture this: you are at work. You are sitting at your desk because your employer doesn't want to promote standing desks; they have come up with some poor excuse like 'it costs too much to change the desks'. (They have not realised that it could cost them more in the long run if you end up off work with a musculoskeletal condition triggered by inactivity.)

Nevertheless, every 60 minutes (which is more realistic than every 30 minutes) you pull away from your desk, sit into a deep squat, then move into a deep lunge with some rotation (picture some sort of yoga pose) and end with a plank position. This takes less than 3 minutes, and then you get straight back into what you were doing – except you are completely revitalised and have both mobile hips and a lively core. It also burns calories. What a wonderful world it would be if this was a normal part of office culture.

For me, I love to find life hacks – especially when it comes to burning fat. When I read that you can burn 12 calories more per minute when you are standing than when you are sitting, I thought, well that's not much. But fat loss is all about small changes leading to big losses.

If, like we said, you sit for 10 hours a day and you just halved that with a standing desk, that's an extra 60 calories burned each day. Over five days a week, that's 300 calories. Over forty-eight weeks of the year, that's 14,400 calories, which equates to 4 lbs of fat. If you were to only change one thing, this would be a starting point – and it doesn't even involve exercising.

Everyone has 24 hours – find time to move

I remember speaking to a dad once. He was sitting on the fence and contemplating whether he had the time to invest in the Super You Project. I always get dads to consider their time if they feel this is an issue when it comes to their health. I have them sit down and consider how much time they truly have to do the things they want to do. I explain to them that time is not a limitless commodity; we are all ageing and moving closer to death (sorry to be morbid). When we calculate how we spend our time, it looks something like this:

If you live to be eighty, you will have 29,200 days (roughly). You'll spend 5,840 of those figuring stuff out until you reach the age of sixteen. We sleep, on average, for 7 hours per day – that's 8,517 days sleeping. That leaves you with 14,843 days. This is always an incredible realisation for the dads I work with, and it certainly was for the dad who was sitting on the fence telling me he didn't have the time to do exercise.

I always get quite preachy when it comes to investing in your health. Your body is here to serve you and can serve you well if you make small investments on a daily basis.

'For God's temple is holy and you are that temple.'[4]

After we have figured out how much time is wasted watching repeated episodes of shows on Netflix, scrolling through phones on social media, or whatever else, we soon discover that there are at least 30 minutes spare in the day to get a little exercise in, even if it's a power walk (this can burn up to 350 calories if it's done at a good pace).

I never train for longer than 30–45 minutes (tops) in one sitting, and I break up disciplines like core strength and mobility across the day in blocks of 5–10 minutes. I use this technique with most of my clients, too. It doesn't have to be about hours spent in the gym. I help change the dads' mindsets to acknowledge this. They then become more productive with the time they do spend exercising. And believe me, as I have already shown with Mac Attack vs Frank the MEP Tank, dads do find time when they want to.

Never skip leg day

And I mean *never*. Why is this an epic mistake? The first reason it's important not to miss leg days is that the pegs we stand on make up an enormous portion of the body, so if you strengthen and condition these muscles hard, you are going to burn some serious calories (which means fat loss).

My clients generally want a leaner torso and a stronger body. Taking this into account, the other benefits of leg days are:

- Better balance

- Increased resilience to injury

- Who wouldn't feel awesome getting stronger and leaner – right?

The second reason it's important not to miss leg days relates to intensity. The legs can endure a lot of physical stress; we can therefore work them harder, for longer periods. An example of this is:

You do twenty press-ups, but if you try to do another twenty with a 15-second rest, you may only manage ten to fifteen. The work rate has stopped. You do twenty lunges. You have a 15-second rest and can manage the same number the second time. The muscles are now larger, as previously mentioned, and take longer to fatigue.

What I often hear is, 'I do a lot of running, and that strengthens my legs,' or, 'I play sport, and that strengthens my legs.' Although these activities will condition your legs, they won't necessarily ensure they get stronger. Achieving stronger legs requires some time spent doing strengthening movements.

'What does a leg session look like?' I hear you say. This depends on your source of information. If you go to bodybuilding websites, the advice will involve splitting the muscles into segments: the quads, glutes, hamstrings (including adductors – inside your legs and hugely neglected) and calves. I tend to forget these and, as a consequence, have calves like an old granny.

Personally, this type of training bores the life out of me, and it certainly doesn't keep my clients' attention. As you may have gathered, I work with busy professional dads who do not have 2 hours a day to spend training each body part separately – although when I set up some challenges for the community, they might take the day off work – yep, they are crazy competitive.

I split my clients' leg days into two categories:

- Deadlift

- Single leg control (lunge, split squat, single leg deadlift, etc)

These movements hit every muscle in the lower body along with placing great demands on the core and upper body. These are referred to as 'functional exercises' because they use multiple joints and multiple muscles, and relate to sporting and daily movements. If those were the only exercises you ever did for the rest of your life, you wouldn't go too far wrong. I encourage each of my clients to do two leg days a week, at different intensities (high and medium). This is usually Monday and Friday for those who have the time during the week, or Friday and Sunday for the 'Weekend Warriors'.

If you take anything from this step, it should be: train your legs, train your legs and, yes, train your legs. They are the beasts that keep you upright. They are where you can make the biggest difference in strength and fat loss.

Do you train hard enough?

As a follow-on from the importance of leg day, I have something to add about maximising results by focusing on training intensity. Picture this:

You go into a gym. You see Frank sitting on the exercise bike reading *Men's Health* magazine and pedalling no faster than 5 km an hour. You see Mike doing bicep curls with 5 kg in the squat rack. Frank is desperate to get in shape for his daughter's beach wedding in Mexico. He's got 20 kg to shift. Mike wants to put some lead back into his pencil by increasing his testosterone levels through strength training (it happens to us all as we get past thirty – testosterone starts to decrease). Looking at what Frank and Mike are doing, do you think they are going to achieve their goals? You guessed it… Nope.

I do get the whole 'something is better than nothing' theory. I too believe in this, to a certain point. But that's more about helping inactive people become active. That has value in itself, but if you want extraordinary results, you must train in an extraordinary way.

Heart rate is a great measure of your intensity during training (as discussed in Step 2). Make no mistake here: I am not promoting always working out like a mad dog. Not at all. Some people choose to ignore this, but it comes back to bite them on the arse. I want my clients to work smarter and get more out of the time they spend doing exercise.

A great example of wasted time in the gym is when I see young men swinging weights to get bigger biceps. Muscles respond best when they are under tension. Without going too geeky on you, the tendons are made of tension-orientated material, meaning they respond best to more stress. Swinging the dumbbells and allowing the tension to release is only short-changing yourself. When you train to increase strength and lean mass, having your mind within the muscle and focusing your attention on that particular area will save you wasting time doing ten reps with no intention at all.

I have found that the best results, in terms of fat loss and lean muscle mass, are obtained by clients when we have focused on 30–45 minutes with absolute intention. If you train, have limited time and have a goal in mind, I urge you to get after it as soon as you step into the training environment. Set your mind to focus before you put on your gym kit. Listen to your favourite '#beastmode' music and kill it. Remind yourself why the hell you started this journey in the first place. Never just go through the motions.

It takes more than motivation to succeed in your fitness goals – it takes discipline.

Coaches' corner

Walking is more powerful than most people realise, and it's a shame that many people all over the world feel like they have to break their back when they first start on their fitness journey. Of course, it's good to build up to training at high intensities, but so often I see clients absolutely smash it for two to three weeks and then burn out – or worse, get injured.

Be aware of the fact that whatever we do, if we are in motion, we are burning calories. You always hear those stories: 'Jimmy never puts weight on and he eats like a horse.' Well, Jimmy never sits still, and he has a physically demanding job on top of walking everywhere he goes. Sit-to-stand desks are quickly becoming an occupational tool for those with lower back pain. The reason is that they allow you to change posture more regularly. There is no single perfect posture; that's a myth. The best posture is moving around on a regular basis.

Once we are ready for some intensity in our training programme, hitting leg day along with some high-intensity sessions will literally melt fat and build muscle. Motion is the lotion.

---

1 Check it out at https://en-gb.facebook.com/ManVerusHorse

2 McCall, P (2017) '6 Things to Know About Non-exercise Activity Thermogenesis'. www.acefitness.org/education-and-resources/lifestyle/blog/6852/6-things-to-know-about-non-exercise-activity-thermogenesis

3 Starrett, K (2016) *Deskbound: Standing Up to a Sitting World*. Las Vegas, NV: Victory Belt.

4 1 Cor. 3:17.

Better Mood, Better Food

Nutrition is the fitness industry's downfall. With every corner they turn, clients are left confused and unsure. There are millions of misleading concepts and thousands of people selling magical potions endorsed by some celebrity bellend. Most people just use the confusion as an excuse to eat like a pig, sit on their arse and do bugger all.

As we've already discussed, my approach is to start with motion. When it comes to food, generally I gear everything around the idea of calories in versus calories out. Understanding energy balance and how to track calories is vital for winning the fat loss battle.

You don't need a meal plan

If I had a pound coin for every time I've been asked, 'Do you write meal plans?' I'd be sipping mojitos with Richard Branson on a sunny beach, surrounded by swimwear models.

When dads approach me, they most often start with that question. They are shocked to the bones when I say to them, point blank: 'No, I have never written a meal plan in my life, and I am not about to start.'

The shock is usually followed by the dad explaining to me that they already know they are guilty of overeating and that their issue is portion control. One dad messaged me one night, told me all his pain points and explained that he was sitting on the fence with regard to joining the online fitness community. I asked him what he needed help with the most. He replied that food was his biggest problem and asked whether I wrote bespoke meal plans.

In my mind, my response was that here was yet another guy who thought this was the answer to all his fitness problems. But like the understanding coach I am, I set him a task. I told him not to change anything at all in his current routine. I messaged back and said, 'All I want you to do is do a power walk every evening for ten days.' His next message said that he would look stupid walking around like that. I replied with a not-so-kind, sharp hit to his heart: 'No, what looks stupid is drinking in the pubs with the lads while bursting out of a shirt in all the wrong places.'

He didn't reply for an hour or so, and I thought I'd cut him too deep. I started to regret being so harsh. Then I got a short message. It said: 'Deal'. After ten days, he had lost 3 kg. He messaged me again: 'I don't need a meal plan, do I?'

If you want ideas for breakfast, lunch and dinner dishes, there are a million books on Amazon. Or, you have access to a billion ideas right there in your pocket. It's called Google. Need I say more?

Calories count, even if you don't count them

There I was, scoffing my third fajita jammed with around 400 calories, thinking, it's OK, I'm walking lots... I'm training twice a day (usually a power walk in the morning and a 30- or 45-minute kettlebell session at lunch). I have earned this. Plus, it's 'healthy food', right?

How naive.

I'd fallen out of the routine of keeping an eye on the calories I was consuming. Even if calories are healthy, they are still calories, and they will be stored as body fat if they are not utilised and torched. I went back to tracking my calories through a food tracker app called MyFitnessPal, and I was shocked to find I was around 200 calories over my recommended calorie allowance on a daily basis. Add this to a weekend binge on roast potatoes and Thai takeaway, and I had been around 1,500 calories over every week, for months.

I went away and created a deficit during the week of 200 calories per day and saw little difference over about six weeks. 'Right, what is going on?' I asked myself.

Every weekend, I was eating a bag of Doritos and a bag of Sports Mix sweets. Just those two things contained an extra 1,600 calories, or thereabouts. My deficit of 1,000 calories (5 x 200) was cancelled out by just those two things – worse, they were creating a 600-calorie overflow. I removed the two snacks from my diet, and the weight started to drop off me.

Is it always that simple? In theory, yes. Calories is always a game of numbers. Do I still count calories? It depends on how things are rolling in my life. If I'm not doing much exercise, I pay more attention to portion size. I have a rough idea of my portion sizes and know that if I am not working out as much, I have to reduce my intake. Calories count, even if you don't count them.

Something else that catches a lot of parents out is the amount of alcohol it is possible to consume at the weekend when we want to chill and take the edge off a busy week. A family member asked me for some advice on his training. His exercise was exactly what he should be doing, and his work rate was intense. He said that, apart from a takeaway here and there, he was spot on with his diet. He ate well all the time and prepped like a boss for himself and his partner, even when he was hungover on a Sunday. The bit about the hangover caught my attention. I asked him how many bottles of beer he tended to drink. He said he drank ten bottles on a Friday night and ten on a Saturday night. Once I told him what was in one bottle of beer (around 140–160 calories), he knew straight away what was stopping him from reaching his fat loss goal – the calories in the beer.

Junk and beer

Sorry about this one, gents, but this is where calories will kill the progress you make during the week if you are not smart about it.

I am not one for having just a couple of beers these days. Being a parent, I can't risk getting the taste for it and then wanting to blow my brains out (responsibilities and all that). My nature (and my genetics – as I mentioned, I come from a family of big drinkers) dictates that I'm an 'all or nothing' drinker.

It's silly of me, and it's something I personally need to work on. I do work on it by taking temptation off the table and mostly not drinking at all. Most people have a lot better self-control when it comes to stuff like this, as I have learned in the Super You Community – most blokes just like a couple of sherbets to chill.

I do know that a lot of my clients like to have a couple on a Friday, Saturday and Sunday. I also have clients who have a couple every night (and still lose body fat, believe it or not). How is this possible?

Ever heard the phrase, 'If it fits your macros'?

This means that, if your overall calorie allowance for the day is 2,500, to lose body fat (if this is your goal – and for most dads over thirty, this is likely to be the case), you need to factor in the couple of beers to your overall consumption. 'So, how many calories are in beer?' I hear you ask.

I touched on this briefly earlier. I'm sorry to be the bearer of bad news, team. These are the calorie counts (roughly):

- Typical pint of beer: 182 calories

- Typical bottle of beer: 142 calories

I don't know about you, but I can polish off ten bottles in one session easily. If I do manage to get a babysitter and take the long-haired admiral out for a few drinks, I will always offset these calories with a beast of a walk and reduce my calories the day after. I advise my clients to manage their alcohol intake in the same way. We have to play it smart and plan for success. If you are one of those dads who drinks a couple of pints most evenings, I advise you to offset the calories with exercise or by not eating as much the next day.

The Offset Rule

I was out with the family one Sunday afternoon and I received a rather bizarre message from a client. It read: 'Dan, I'm at a birthday party, and I really want to have a beer and some cake.' My first thought was that it was a weird combination. But hell, who am I to judge?

This dad had been in my community for around six weeks and had lost about 10 kg. He was doing amazingly well. Then it started to unfold *why* he was doing so well. I asked him if he had watched any of my videos about eating *what* you want, just not *as much* as you want. The videos cover the importance of protein and the total daily energy expenditure (TDEE) magic number.

He said that he hadn't. Alarm bells started to ring. He asked what TDEE was, and then went on to tell me that he'd never tracked the amount of protein he ate or the calories he ingested. I had to explain that TDEE was the number of calories that he needs to survive (to perform basic bodily functions along with the activities of daily living) and that if he wanted to lose body fat in the long term (lifestyle changes), he needed to eat 15–20% less than his TDEE number for steady and safe fat loss. I also explained that if he was restricting his foods and was on rigid diet programmes, it could lead to elevated hormone levels that would push him to overeat and relapse.

He was shocked and embarrassed that he had not watched any of the videos. I reassured him that having a beer and some cake was not a problem as long as he used the Offset Rule. He asked what the Offset Rule was. As you can imagine, by now I was wondering how he had got this far. I explained that if you want to eat and overindulge on certain occasions, you need a plan to work the extra calories off somehow or under-eat the next day – but without sacrificing your daily protein goal.

He was bamboozled. There was a pause. Then he asked, 'What's my protein goal again?'

I explained that, during exercise periods, it is advised that we should eat anything from 1.4 grams to 2.4 grams of protein per kilogram of bodyweight. I highlighted the fact that this helps with maintaining lean body mass during the fat loss phase. The lightbulb finally switched on, and he was over the moon that he could eat the cake and drink the beer. I did have to ask him at that point what the hell he had been eating. It turned out to be a 'fish and rice cake' diet he had seen on YouTube.

Eating the leftovers

No one likes food to go to waste, especially when it's fish fingers and chips. (Or is that just me?) That said, you know kids – they are always going to leave food because they want to leave room for dessert. Take my daughter, for example. As she is getting older, wiser and cheekier, her habits in relation to finishing her food have changed drastically. No longer will she eat all her potatoes during our Sunday roast; she is leaving room for the chocolate pudding. Being a roast potato lover, I find it difficult to let them go to waste.

The way you need to think about leftovers is this: if eating leftover food is a regular occurrence (the opportunity crops up every day in our house), these extra calories are going to have an impact on your waistline. As you will have gathered by now, I speak about calories all the time because this is what we need. We need to cut the BS and stick to hard facts. They count, even if you don't count them. *They count, even if you don't count them.* I will say this until I am blue in the face.

Yes, food waste is a shame, certainly. There are many people in the world who go without. But it's not your responsibility to eat all the leftovers just because your mum told you that good food should not go to waste. These sorts of lifelong habits and ingrained behaviours are probably the most common things that sabotage fat loss success. I know this is a hard one to break. All I will say is, think of your waistline when deciding whether or not to let food go to waste.

Shopping on an empty stomach

I don't have much experience of this these days, as we do our shopping online. It's so much easier and saves a lot of time – which is hugely valuable as a parent, right? That said, back in the day, if I stepped into Tesco on a Friday afternoon having not eaten anything since breakfast, I would be straight to the Doritos and sweets. Don't get me wrong, having this type of food is OK if it fits within your calorie allowance for that day (if you are training to lose body fat, that is). However, I would eat my daily calories before I even had a chance to pay for the rest of the shopping.

The solution? Before you do your shopping, make sure you eat something that fits in better with your fitness goals. A technique that a dad I was working with one-to-one found useful was checking the calories he had left in his daily allowance. If he had lots left on the table, then I would always advise him to go to the hot deli or the delicatessen for something high protein and with more nutritional value – this would help towards his protein goals.

Preparation is key

I saw a post on Instagram once from a company selling ready-prepared meals containing the right amounts of calories and macros, etc to meet your nutritional requirements. Wow, I thought. Someone had hit the market with perfect timing. Although many people won't have the money to buy meals from these types of incredible food prep companies, I thought it was a wicked idea – certainly for busy parents. But if most of us haven't got the readies for this – we're parents; things like this are a luxury, right? – what can we do to achieve the same thing?

I cook with similar ingredients on most days. I just change the way my food is cooked. I make sure I have plenty of veggies and always have lots of fruit. This is essential for any type of long-term muscle building and maintenance of a healthy body. Although I am a huge advocate of the 'eat what you want, just not as much as you want' approach, there are still some fundamentals when it comes to food that we need to be on top of. Eating plenty of fruit and veggies is definitely one of those. I also tend to cook extra in the evening so that I have food to take to work the next day. This works better for my partner and me. We are both working parents, so to put 2–3 hours aside on a Sunday to prepare food for the week is, for us, unrealistic. I'm not saying it is not possible, just that it wouldn't work for us.

My plan is to only have wholefoods in my home so that I don't have the opportunity to indulge in foods that are not conducive to my fitness goals. While I'm flexible in my nutritional game plan, I still play it smart, especially throughout the week. I often create a calorie deficit (burning more calories than I put in) over the week. My breakfast and lunches are similar on most days, along with my snacks. I keep a close eye on my protein goal. The rest, I'm flexible with.

Food prep is more about routine and perception. Lots of people will want to eat different foods every day. For me, that would just mean I had to make more choices. Like I said above, I cut those down by eating the same things during the day most of the week (I'm ex-military, remember – drills and routine come naturally).

My relationship with food through the week is that it is fuel and necessary for me to function as a content human being. An example of my daily food:

- Breakfast – needs to be quick, so I have smoothies that contain oats, milk and frozen fruit. It takes literally 2 minutes to make one of these, and it has about 600–700 calories.

- Mid-morning snack – protein yogurt with honey and oats, about 400–500 calories.

- Lunch – usually last night's leftovers. This will be around 500–600 calories.

- Dinner – this varies, but it always involves rice or tortilla wraps with either chicken or fish and veggies. I prepare these in different spices and sauces and dinner comes out around 700–800 calories.

That is as difficult as I make my meal preparation. If I want new ideas, that's what Google is for.

Coaches' corner

Food intake is the aspect of fitness that most blokes think they have a problem with. It's not. The problem is their relationship with food. They think they need a meal plan, but they will probably never stick to it, and it will sit in their inbox for eternity, gathering cyber-dust. The best guidance I can give to any dad starting the fitness and fat loss journey is to understand that calories matter. It is worth downloading a calorie tracker and starting to get to grips with the amount of energy that is in the food you eat. This is vital for any success in fat loss.

Mostly, the issue of consumption is about awareness of the small things – all those factors that initially trip up everyone I've worked with on their journey to lose body fat. Giving them the hard facts that they need to track their calories for a period of time until they know how much they are actually consuming is fundamental. When I ask dads what they think they need to do to sort out their food intake, most of them already know the answer: cut down on the junk, increase their fruit and veg intake, and keep their protein intake high.

Binger Vs Consistency Ninja

There are some subtle differences between those who are successful in fat loss (the ninjas) and those who are not (the bingers). The binger will come out all guns blazing. He will write a long list of goals and will expect that these will be complete within a month. Typically, he will hit the gym hard for the first week of the month and tell everyone he is on a 'health kick'. He will burn up to 5,000 calories through exercise alone that week. The week after that, he will hit it hard, but not *as* hard. He will burn 4,000 calories through exercise. The week after that… The binger is beat.

Injuries will start to creep in, and the wind in his sail is depleted. He will barely manage two sessions in the week and will feel the urge to overeat due to his rapid fat loss and his hormones being all over the place from the excessive training. His hunger levels will be through the roof as a result of heavily restricted dieting. He will burn 1,000 calories through exercise that week. By the fourth week, the poor man is AWOL. He's missing in action. He's nowhere to be seen. His total calorie-burn over the month is 10,000, which equates to 1.5 kg of body fat. He never wants to go through that ever again.

As for the ninja, he will set out at a steady pace. He will write down one goal and will accept that it could take three to six months to achieve. He will typically hit the gym with consistency for the first week of the month, burning up to 2,500 calories through exercise alone. The week after, he will hit it at a similar pace – but this week he will already be feeling stronger. He will burn 3,000 calories through exercise this week. By the third week, the ninja will be beating down the door to get his exercise fix. The motivation is like an inferno. He's like a mad dog. Any injuries will have started to disappear, and the wind will be fully in his sail. He will manage a little more and will feel the urge to add something else. By being flexible with his diet, management of hunger levels will be spot on. He will burn 3,500 calories through exercise this week. By the fourth week, he will move into complete #beastmode and burn 5,000 calories.

His total calorie-burn for the month is 14,500, which equates to 2 kg of fat. He cannot wait for the next month.

The following case studies illustrate the difference in detail.

THE CONSISTENCY NINJA – 168 NOT OUT

Cricket has never been a game I watch religiously, but I do admire it when a sportsperson does something remarkable that leaves the audience in admiration.

Back in 2004, West Indies batman Brian Lara shocked the England Cricket Team with his exceptional effort of 400 runs not out. Scoring a century (100 runs) is impressive enough. To not only triple this score but quadruple it... that is just immense. This shows the type of focus needed to achieve greatness. You have to be consistent in every aspect of the sport, both on and off the field.

I see fitness and fat loss in the same way. When I started the Super You Community, I worked with one dad who was adamant he couldn't stick to something for more than thirty days. We chatted about everything that he had tried before, from multi-level marketing products to enrolling in charity events to keep him interested; he said he always managed to steer away from the goal. I told him I would make a pact with him, and that I would do a minimum of a 30-minute power walk every single day of the year if he did it with me. He made the deal.

For the first thirty days, it was easy for both of us. October is usually fairly quiet for parents. November came along, and towards the back end of the month, family functions along with work Christmas parties started to sneak in. I messaged him on social media every time I saw that he'd been for a couple of beers with the boys, or that he'd had a family weekend filled with booze and great food. He messaged me back once around late December time to say that he might not fulfil the pact he'd made with me.

I couldn't see him do this to his winning streak. By this point, he was close to 100 days not out. He had managed almost 100 days of physical activity. Although the choice to get out and get it done was becoming harder, I kept reassuring him that consistency is rewarded with increased fitness. He dug deep over the festive period and got out in the cold wet nights every single day. January came around, and he was over the moon that he'd managed to stay on track with just one thing.

His feedback was that, although he may have overindulged in food while partying in December, staying on track with just a little exercise made it easy to up the pace when January came around. I told him that it's easier to stay on the horse than it is to get back on, meaning that even if what you're doing is something small, your choice is strengthening the decision pathways in your brain. This is hugely important when motivation is low and discipline has to take its place.

He finally ended his amazing streak in March, after 168 consecutive days of physical activity. Not quite a full year, but an awesome achievement nonetheless. This, for me, shows what we can achieve when we manage our time and make fitness a priority rather than a luxury. This dad works shifts, has two children under the age of ten and is very much involved in family life. To this day, he continues to be consistent with his exercise, as he's discovered that consistency builds momentum, and momentum got him results – like running the fastest 5 km and 10 km he had ever run in his life. In the Super You Community, he has earned the official title of 'Consistency Ninja'.

THE BINGER – INSANITY OR CHANGE

I have been told many times that you can't help everyone, but it isn't in my nature to accept that. No matter who I work with, if they have come to me for help, I will believe that they are going to put the work in.

As a physical trainer (PT), I get to meet people from all walks of life, but one dad in particular stands out. He was a bit 'big time' and had a loud mouth, which I thought might be a front. That said, after a few weeks his pace didn't slow when it came to fitness. The idea of 'start with one thing' didn't seem to resonate with him. He went from zero to 100 miles per hour within the first few weeks.

I thought there was no way he'd be able to keep the pace up. He was doing 2-hour workouts almost every day (considering he'd told me he didn't have time, that is epic).

It was a worry for me, as I knew he was carrying a lot of weight and that going at such a pace could risk injury. After about a month, he had lost around 9 kg. He was over the moon.

He was well and truly on the horse… But he was riding too fast. He had a holiday on the horizon. He was yet another dad who had not read any of the emails I'd sent with tips (such as the Offset Rule) to prepare for things like holidays and special occasions.

He was stressed.

He went away on holiday. As I'm sure you've guessed, it all fell apart. He came fully off the horse. He decided that, because he'd worked hard for the past six weeks, it wasn't necessary to do even just one thing while he was away. He was off the horse and didn't look likely to get back on.

We had a few words, and I pointed him in the right direction. I sent him links to the videos and hoped he'd take the advice on board. Boom. He went from zero to 100 miles per hour again.

He lost some weight but the progress was slow, and he was getting frustrated. He was drinking heavily at the weekend and overindulging in junk food but convincing himself it wouldn't have an impact because of the effort he was putting into his fitness sessions. He had hit a point where he was not going to lose any more fat unless he changed other aspects of his lifestyle. I explained to him that how he was spending his weekends was sabotaging all his good work, and that I'd seen this with many of my clients. I hoped that this time, it would sink in... But it didn't.

Einstein once said that insanity is doing the same thing again and expecting something to change. This dad is a clear example of how bingeing affects your results in the long term.

Focus on the necessary – and be consistent

Being ex-military and playing one of the fastest-paced sports in the world, I was used to going for it all the time. I had the 'go hard or go home' mentality and have the scars to show for it. The thing is, what did that mindset actually achieve? Yes, I managed to put my mind and body through some trauma and come out the other side with some huge achievements – but did that mean that I always had to go for it in a workout environment?

My injuries as I reached my thirties were becoming unmanageable, and it was looking like I would need more surgery on my knee and ankle. I wasn't a happy chap. I started to do some research into training with kettlebells and, as is my nature, I searched for the best people in the industry to learn from. There is no other way, in my opinion. I came across a philosophy that originated in Russia, and which made me strip my training back to invest in a basic fundamental programme.

Although I am consistent and never miss a training day, I have always struggled to stick with just one programme for a long period of time, and I used to get distracted with what everyone else was doing – I am only human.

But I stuck rigidly to this programme – no more and no less – and practised daily. At first it drove me insane. I cursed and said, 'This programme isn't doing anything for me.' I felt like I was losing fitness. I felt like I was losing muscle mass. It was all internal mind games.

I managed to stick to it for twelve whole weeks. Twelve whole weeks of just five basic kettlebell exercises. After this time, I thought it was a good idea to put my new skills in remaining consistent to one programme to the test. To my surprise, my one-rep maximum (lifting for maximum effort for one repetition) in deadlift had gone from 180 kg to 200 kg without me having lifted anything more than a 32-kg kettlebell. The movement during the deadlift was so slick that I had managed to gain 20 kg in the beast of all lifts.

After twelve weeks, I'd decreased my body fat percentage (I was eating well during this time) and increased muscle tone. As I said, sometimes it's all in your head. What did this tell me? It told me that we must stay consistent and focus on training the things that matter. It told me that if you want to see change, you have to let go of the old thinking that is keeping you where you are now.

Being consistent is being obedient to the process. From the Russian principles, I learned that strength is the master of all fitness disciplines. From strength, we can build mobility (moving more freely), stability (controlling movement better, which is important to prevent injury), and conditioning (building an engine to move with purpose and increase our work capacity). If we have a foundation of strength, this means that we can go for longer and endure more in other aspects of fitness. Strength is trial and error. Try a dose – **if** it's too little, do more; if it's too much, do less.

Am I saying that everyone needs to do basic programmes? I'm saying that everyone wants to try out the shiny new things outside the box before they have mastered the things already in the box. I am saying that you should assess what matters to you. If you want to take your fitness seriously and see results, you must be consistent. These days, I write all my programmes with this in mind. I focus on training for everyday life and maximising the movements – like the deadlift and lunge – that will benefit other movements in everyday activities.

Coaches' corner

Having worked with a variety of people in my many years in the fitness industry, the difference between those who succeed in their goals and those who don't is clear to see. The clients who choose to master the basics, take everything in their stride and remain consistent always reap the benefits. The clients who are more up and down than the stock market often swing from one programme to another and never find the benefits they are looking for because they don't stick to anything long enough to create any results.

Bingeing is a habit that can only lead to failure because there is no consistency; you're either high and very motivated or low and can't find any motivation at all. The consistency ninja is a clear example of what it takes to make those hard decisions and how those choices get easier when you make them consistently every day. When we stick to something long enough, we are bound to see rewards.

Consistency builds momentum. Momentum leads to success.

Treat Yourself As You Would Treat Your Nan

As parents, something that tends to get overlooked is our own health and well-being. For most, it is an afterthought and something they postpone. You know the score, 'When the kids go to school in a couple of years, I'll get my gym kit out again.' The thing is, most of the time this never happens, and it gets harder by the year to get back on the horse. I hear it all the time from hard-working dads who are doing their best to provide for their families. They say, 'I don't know where to start,' or, 'I thought I was past all this health and fitness stuff.'

Sorry to get on my soapbox about this one, but health is wealth – unfortunately, most take it for granted until they have a health scare or something happens that literally gets them off their arse to move. Dads become so good at looking after everyone else's health, they neglect their own – and usually they feel unhappy and discontent as a consequence. The way I put it to all my clients is: 'How would you treat your nan's health?'

The American dream

I love my nanna. My mum said that I always wanted to be close to her when I was young. Growing up in sunny Hull, I could be quite a handful. My behaviour as a child wasn't the best, and I often found myself apologising to my mum and nan. When I finally left home to join the steak and gravy (the

Navy, for those not accustomed to Cockney slang), I had a dream of taking my mum and nan to Memphis. We are all massive Elvis Presley fans, and throughout my childhood we listened to him whenever we were in the car.

In 2009, I had the opportunity to go on tour to the Falkland Islands for six months. There isn't much to do on the island for servicemen and women, apart from either getting pissed or getting shredded in the awesome gym facilities down there. This tour gave me a healthy bank balance (nothing to spend my money on, you see), and the opportunity to finally repay my mum and nan's kindness while I was growing up.

I booked us a jet-set holiday to the US. I didn't just book Memphis. Oh no. 'What the hell,' I thought, 'We only live once.' I booked New York and Las Vegas to top the trip off.

At the time, my nan was about to turn seventy and my mum was fifty years old. I felt totally responsible for my nan, as I had taken her out of the safe and comfortable environment she was used to, but I knew I was capable of fulfilling her care needs. I thought about every aspect of what it takes to stay alive; not just to stay alive, but to be content and happy. I thought about it all from my nan's perspective. Every day, I made sure we had breakfast at a decent time, I made sure we had lunch, and I made a big fuss at dinner.

What I learned from that trip was that if I could treat myself with that same respect and uphold the same responsibility for my own routine, a few things would happen:

- I would eat regular and wholesome foods and not overfeed myself

- I would drink the amount of water needed for me to function well as a human being

- I would sleep for at least 7 hours a day, to ensure attentiveness (sometimes a problem for parents)

Responsibility for personal well-being can fall by the wayside when we have others to think about and look after, especially as a parent. But if you are not functioning well, how can you give someone else your best? The dads I work with are amazed at how much more engaged they are with family activity and how energised they feel at the weekend after doing exercise for just a few weeks.

Taking care of yourself is essential if you're going to show up every day and be the best son, dad, brother, grandad, husband, partner, boyfriend, friend – or any of the many other roles we play in life. Not always looking after ourselves is something we are all guilty of, and it is something I will challenge you on.

Take care of yourself. Find time in your day and treat yourself as you would treat your nan.

BREATHING SPACE

I was about to see a patient once who was going for spinal surgery. My mind was challenging me to just have a brief chat and reassure him that after the surgery we could start working together properly. But what exercise would I be able to do with someone with so many functional limitations that they could barely walk?

When he came through the door, I could see the pain in his eyes. As soon as I saw him, I wanted to help him in any way possible. I got him to do the 6-minute walk test used with patients with chronic obstruction pulmonary disease. I thought it might be appropriate to just get him moving in some way. He covered 0.19 km in 6 minutes. That's not even 200 metres in 6 minutes. The man was in severe pain.

I asked him to get into a position that he was comfortable in. He got onto his hands and knees. Once he was in a comfortable position, I got him to do some deep lateral breathing (filling out the stomach, flaring the ribs outwards and relaxing the shoulders), counting from seven to one during the inhale and counting from one to seven on the exhale, with a pause for a count of three at the bottom and at the top of the breath. We did this for ten repetitions. Then he got up and had a little walk and did it again. We repeated the process for about 20 minutes.

I then asked him to complete the 6-minute walk test again – he managed to double his distance. By taking control of his breathing, we had reduced his stress levels. This patient was highly stressed, feeling anxiety about the operation and also about the constant pain in his back. He was all over the place with his mental hygiene.

I promote the breathing technique outlined above to deal with stress. I usually start with 2–3 minutes total and build up from there. Try it. Having used these sorts of techniques for many years, I know that bringing that level of attention into your life can be a real game changer. Breathing like this can give you some thinking space, so valuable in the stressful environments we live in today. Can you imagine how much patience the guy going for surgery had to have once he was home? Not being able to get involved with running the house was incredibly frustrating. He carried on using this simple technique after his surgery. Giving him that bit of breathing space worked wonders, and he carried on with the simple system as he found it chilled him out.

Breathing is a way to deal with stressful environments – there is plenty of science to support this.

Finding balance

I get it. We all are hooked on the belief that fitness and health is all about shredded abs and big round booties. But is that *really* what we are trying to achieve?

Back in the day, when I was highly impressionable and easily influenced, I attended a neuro-linguistic programming (NLP) seminar. It had its good and bad points. One of the good points I took away was about 'chunking down' or 'chunking up'. This was a process whereby you would be asked to articulate questions to find the bigger picture of what you were trying to achieve – the overall 'why?'.

When I work with dads, more often than not there is a bigger picture as to why they want to lose weight or build muscle, though these are usually the things they mention first. Their reasons for wanting to work with me usually stem from a deeper place, but I find that their physical goals are something that gets the conversation started. Once we have scratched the surface, we start to get to the real reasons they have sought help with their lifestyle.

A phrase I hear quite often is, 'I feel a little unbalanced.' To me, this means they are here to work with me on a lot more than getting fitter and losing weight. Balance means different things to different people. Here are a few things to consider:

1. Mindset – taking charge of your breathing has been scientifically proven to increase your productivity and attentiveness. This will help to create a balanced life during both work and play.

2. Movement – moving well is essential to improving and maintaining your quality of life and balancing the mental and the physical.

3. Munch – managing your choices, understanding portion size and mastering your cravings will assist in achieving balanced nutrition.

4. Sleep – sleeping peacefully, with a balanced daily and nightly routine, creates good sleep hygiene, which is vital for health.

5. Connection – making time to connect with your loved ones and be completely present in their company will create balanced relationships.

6. Play and adventure – having fun and de-loading by taking time out to let loose and relax will create balance between work and the rest of your life.

7. A wider perspective – thinking more about how we can help others and our communities to feel enriched and fulfilled creates balance between looking inwards and looking outwards.

It's unrealistic to expect to always be at 100% in each of these areas. But we can aim to have an understanding of each, and to assess our situation in these aspects of our life if everything is feeling a little too chaotic and this is affecting our general health.

If you review these aspects of balance, I expect you might find something to work on to improve your situation.

WHY SO SERIOUS?

When I hit my thirties and had my daughter, I felt overwhelmed with responsibility, a sense that the buck stopped with me.

I could feel an element of seriousness creeping into my life. It was weird because I had never taken anything too seriously before – but now I had to take care of another human being. Now I had to make sure I could provide. It started to suck the joy out of me. It feels bad to admit that.

I thought I always had to act grown-up. Even though she was a baby, I thought joking around would mean I wasn't projecting a persona of authority. I asked other dads about this, and they admitted that they struggled with the same thing. The 'end of happiness' was how one dad phrased it.

I didn't believe it. I get that, as dads, we worry about everything more, of course – and certainly while our children are still under our roof. But the 'end of happiness'?

I graded my happiness on a scale of one to ten – I was a five. I felt guilty about that. How could I have the most beautiful daughter in the world, a beautiful partner, good health and a great job and be a five?

I started to assess how often I was spending time with my loved ones and my friends. I asked myself: how much time do I spend having adventures? Playing music? Getting out into the great outdoors?

I began to panic. I was becoming so serious that I had stopped having fun. Life can't be serious all the time. Thinking we have to play the authoritarian at home and getting too involved in making money will mean we forget to build a life.

We may be smashing the deadlines at work, beating our 10 km times on the road, lifting heavy weights and looking super-ripped – but even the strongest of us will eventually burn out. If we are distant from the rest of the world and have no social life, these goals we achieve will come and go, and when we turn around to see who is with us and nobody is there, are they going to be worth it?

Coaches' corner

Considering how we treat others and treating ourselves the same way is a reminder that our own health is not a luxury and that it needs care and attention. Moving on from 'one thing' to the next goal may involve taking charge of your breathing, especially if you work in a stressful environment. It is certainly a life hack that I have found has major benefits for both clients and patients.

Balance in life is sometimes hard to define. Once you can identify what things you need to balance, you will be empowered to take charge of the aspects of your life that may be out of sync. Making connections and having fun are things that a lot of us postpone. But we forget that bittersweet truth – that we are all going to die one day, so bring some balance to your perspective, and make the most of every precious day.

The Gremlins Of Fat Loss

Gremlins are the little annoying things that we can't quite get a hold on. These are the little problems that dads I work with often present later, once we have worked together for a few months. Most dads are not aware of these at first, so they end up damaging their results.

It's painful to watch, especially after they have spent a few months in the Super You Community and I have talked to them about the fact that their current approach to fitness and fat loss isn't getting them the results they want. It can't be, or they wouldn't be seeking out someone like me in the first place. Often, dads will take the guidance on board for about a week and expect instant and long-lasting results. But it just doesn't work that way.

For some specific fitness goals, there can be instant results. I have helped someone improve their core endurance in just seven days. I have helped guys drop two jean sizes in five days. But for those results to be long-lasting, the relevant practices must be adhered to for longer periods of time. They must become a lifestyle.

Here are some of the gremlins that snap away at all the dads I work with.

Overcomplicating things and making excuses

What holds dads back most of the time is the excuses they make after they have started.

Excuse: 'My partner likes my love handles, so I best not get in too good shape.'

Truth: Your partner is stroking their insecurities and doesn't want you to run off with the next-door neighbour when you become a dad god after ditching the dad bod.

Excuse: 'I have had two children, so I'll never get fit again. Those days are long gone.'

Truth: Now it's even more important to become fitter than ever. If you want your children to be fit, you need to show them how it's done.

Excuse: 'I have the fat gene – it's in the family.'

Truth: You are what you repeatedly do; genes don't necessarily have to express themselves. I am a good example of this. The majority of my family are severely overweight or obese, yet I have managed to stay slim and lean most of my life.

I will call people out on all these excuses, all day long. They are just crutches that people feel safe holding onto.

Thinking too much about the consequences of being healthy and fit can be daunting. Let me put it like this: if you are used to being known to your friends as 'Fat Phil', what will you been known as if you get fit? Identity crisis? No, they'll just call you 'Fit Phil'. As silly as this sounds, if you are defined by your problem, your mind will find it hard to let go of old characteristics when you change. Change is uncomfortable. Limiting beliefs like this are powerful, so much so that they can prevent you from moving forward and achieving your goals.

Find a quiet place and write down all the things that seem complicated to you in the pursuit of your goals. Next to each complication, write a solution, how you can overcome it. For example:

Complication: I don't seem to have time to work out.

Questions to ask yourself:

- Can I get up early in the morning?

- Do I have to watch *Game of Thrones* every night?

- What do I do at lunchtime?

- Can I go for a power walk?

- Can I do 20 minutes of press-ups and lunges?

Using this type of thinking promotes more useful ideas. The problems you thought were complicated are just excuses getting in the way of you becoming the best you can be.

Running is not the best route to fat loss

Possibly one of the biggest misconceptions within the fat loss industry – and one held by most of the clients and patients I have worked with – is 'I need to run to lose weight'. This thought process is limiting. There is more than one way to skin a cat, as the saying goes.

Working for many years with the British Army in a rehabilitation clinic helping injured soldiers get back to full fitness has certainly given me insight into this myth. Many people think that running is the best route to fat loss. Notice how I keep saying fat loss and not weight loss – they are different.

I always promote fat loss rather than weight loss, because maintaining lean muscle mass is essential for staying strong to cope with the activities of daily living (lifting, stairs, moving, etc).

Beliefs like 'we are born to run' have been around for years. But I'm not convinced we are. One thing is for certain though: we are born to walk, and to move from place to place. Yes, running can help with weight loss (OK, it can help with fat loss, too), but my point is that it isn't the be all and end all.

A fair few of the dads are initially resistant to my principle of starting with a power walk. Some of those dads may be carrying up to 30 kg more weight than their body shape needs. What tends to happen, nine times out of ten, is that they will ignore my guidance, think that they are twenty-one again, and go for a 10 km run. The next day, they won't be able to walk and will message me to tell me how tight their shins are, or that their knees are playing up.

A little exercise here. Pick a 20-kg weight and walk with it for 1 minute. Do you see and feel my point? If you are overweight and looking to get back into running, I would highly advise you do this gradually. I use a 'return to running' programme with the dads I work with and have used it for many years with patients returning from injury. You start by walking for 4.5 minutes and then run gently for 30 seconds. Each week, you reduce the walk by 30 seconds and increase the run by 30 seconds. You do this for 30 minutes in total each session. If, like me, you have some old injuries that are provoked by too much impact, walking combined with strength training is golden for fat loss.

While I am on this subject, let's define walking. With the power walking I am referring to, you need to be out of breath. Not bleeding from the eyeballs, but enough to get sweaty. I started at a pace (measured using an app called Runkeeper) of around 10 min/km, and I do the same with my clients. To start with, keep this pace up over a distance of around 3.2 km (which should take around 30–40 minutes). Every week, do your best to shave 5 seconds off your time. Needless to say, after six months of working with some of my clients, they are doing 8 min/km and have dropped some significant body fat.

An unsupportive partner

This is not me being a prick – this is me bringing it to your attention that sometimes others might want you to stay as you are because, if you change, they might have to as well. What has been strange to witness with some of the guys I have worked with is that their partners have been unsupportive (often in an indirect way) of their fitness goals.

What do I mean by 'indirect'? Well, they don't come out and say, 'I'm not happy with you trying to get fitter, stronger and leaner so you can perform better as a father due to the positive mindset this gives you as a human being.' But there will be subtle things going on. I've heard stories of partners piling my clients' plates up with food when it is their turn to cook, knowing this means unnecessary calories, even though portion size has been discussed.

I've heard stories of partners making it almost impossible for my clients to train by guilt-tripping them into feeling that it makes them a more supportive person to stay in the living room, sit on their arse watching *EastEnders* and pick at a bowl of Doritos.

Our partners have more power over our decisions than we often realise, so it's worth becoming aware of whether your partner is supporting you in your quest for fitness or sabotaging your progress. If it is the latter, it's time to call a relationship meeting, work out why this is happening, and get your partner onside – possibly by getting them involved. In fact, many of the dads I work with get their entire families involved. For me, putting fitness at the centre of family life can only be a good thing. If dads and kids are doing the fitness thing, our partners are more likely to shift their mindsets too.

The Chinese bamboo analogy

In Chinese culture, it is believed that success is like a bamboo plant. In the first year, it needs water, sunshine and good soil, and you won't see a shoot. In the second year, it needs the same. You won't see progress, but the seed still requires care and attention. In the third year, most have given up on the seed and lost faith that one day they will see the bamboo rise above the soil. Those who have been patient and continued providing sunlight and water still don't see any progress after the fourth year. Then, in the fifth year, like a miracle, the bamboo grows up to 80 feet in just six weeks.

This is a perfect example of the patience it takes to build and maintain solid, lifelong fitness. One question that all people looking to achieve any type of fitness goal should ask themselves is: how long do you think it will take to achieve this?

I can tell you now that eight-week programmes and short fixes just do not cut it for promoting permanent behaviour change. We are setting people up to fail when we have no follow-up, no community, no accountability. Just look at the state of the Western world. We have so many quick fixes, yet people are more unwell, are buying bigger clothes and are sadder than ever before.

What is happening?

Yes, amazing things can be achieved within short periods, but will those changes last? Are they sustainable? I completely agree that short-term programmes are a good kick-start, but are they a kick-start into consistent, positive and long-lasting behaviour?

As I mentioned earlier, I once worked at the most famous women's boot camp in the UK. There were several women there who had been more than once. I asked them, 'How come you are here again?' and they mostly replied, 'It's a great kick-starter.' But needing 'a great kick-starter' *every year* should set alarm bells ringing if they turn up looking the same as they did the year before and struggling once again with exercise. The 'binger' problem comes to mind here – or sometimes people are just not equipped with a good solid process and tools that last a lifetime.

What is it in their behaviour that is leading them to fall out of a good routine and return to poor habits, meaning they end up back at boot camp for a quick fix? If it's the community the boot camp offers that they need, I get it. Meeting new people with the same goal and a similar mindset is great. If it's lack of motivation, we need to talk, as motivation must grow into discipline for long-term success.

If any of this resonates with you, ask yourself what you can do to change this right now. I don't mean to be all doom and gloom. I just feel it is important to highlight the gremlins we face so that we can overcome them. I want you to understand what it takes and that patience will pay off in the end. Patience is like every other principle I have discussed – you have to practise and dig deep when progress is slow. If you want long-lasting results, you must treat fitness as a lifelong journey, and have something meaningful to focus on. I often suggest to my clients that they get involved in charity events, and obviously my fitness community will help with this too. These things support, reinforce and make bulletproof people's beliefs that being healthy is better than being unhealthy – and believe me, there are people who believe they are better off unhealthy.

Coaches' corner

The gremlins outlined above will probably resonate with most people who read this, one or two more than others, but I am sure that at least one will be nibbling away at your progress.

The thing is, once we are aware of the gremlin, we can put into place a plan to overcome that particular barrier. As you have probably noticed, I don't overcomplicate things. This takes any confusion off the table and allows my clients to focus on their goal, whatever that may be.

You don't want to put yourself in situations where there are too many options, as this leads to decision burnout, which in turn leads to poor choices (think about being in a restaurant). Running might not be the best option for those who are carrying a bit of extra weight, but that isn't a problem as there are many other fitness activities that can help you achieve your fat loss or fitness goals.

Consider involving your partner as you get more immersed in the fitness journey. It makes life a lot easier. I took this to the next level and convinced my partner to become a PT in the Royal Navy after she had our daughter – yes, I am extreme, as I'm sure you have noticed.

Being aware of the time it takes to be successful at anything in life removes the lethal disappointment of unrealistic expectations. Be realistic in all of your goals.

Plateau Isn't A Place In Greece – Nor Is It A Place In Fat Loss

A long-term hitch I run into with many of my clients is the dreaded plateau. You get an email that reads: 'Hey, I have stopped losing weight, what the hell, man?' This is the reply I send: 'Plateau is not a place in Greece – nor is it a place in fat loss.' They will often laugh at first, then ask me to go into a little more detail. I explain that plateaus simply don't exist in fitness or fat loss; it's a case of finding marginal gains.

To be frank, if you are 20–30 kg overweight, you have a lot to lose before this might become a problem. Most of the time, in the early days fat loss is straightforward: it's about moving more and eating less. In some cases, it might be a little more complicated due to life stresses. Maybe the management of boredom eating or comfort eating might play a part, but once these are brought to your attention, there is an opportunity to change. Very rarely, an underlying medical condition may be preventing progress in fat loss, but as a rule, just getting the basics right should take you towards your desired result.

You have to think of fat loss as a numbers game; it involves giving and taking. As you will be aware by now, fat loss is about mindset. Knowing the difference between a drive to eat and genuine hunger is what leads most people to successful fat loss. The difficulty is that it takes effort, and you have to be ruthless with paying attention to what you are eating for the first few months, until you are confident you know your portion sizes inside out.

I have learned a few lessons over the years from seeing people who feel like they have plateaued and who need to be mindful of what may be causing this.

CHANGE YOUR TDEE WHENEVER YOU LOSE 4–6 KG

A dad came to me who wanted to lose 15 kg. He was going on holiday with his family and said that if I could help him fit into the shirts he wore on a holiday he'd had pre-kids, he would be mega-grateful. I accepted the challenge. I explained everything that needed to happen for him to be achieve his goal. He was totally onside.

A few weeks into the programme, he was killing it; he was 3 kg down and the weight was steadily shifting. He hit 5 kg of fat loss and then stayed there for about two weeks.

He was distressed and almost turning on me, like a snake ready to bite my head off. His so-called plateau had really got to him.

'Why have I stopped losing weight, Dan? I am doing everything you said to do.' I could feel his frustration. 'Right. Have you adjusted your TDEE?' I replied. I always lead with this question. He hadn't.

Let me explain this to you. This guy lost 5 kg by consuming 3,000 calories a day. After he'd taken exercise into account, that put him in a calorie deficit of around 500 calories per day. Eventually, he would be at a weight where the food he was eating would maintain his current weight.

Your TDEE is calculated based on your gender, age, weight, height and activity level. Notice how weight is included here? When this guy lost 5 kg, that was a significant enough change for him to need to adjust the TDEE to lose more weight.

This is where I start when any of my clients come to me with, 'I've hit a plateau.'

Secret eating

There used to be a programme on TV that followed people with a secret camera to capture every single moment of their life and highlight where they were going wrong when it came to their nutritional game plan. It was entertaining, and it used to shock me how many people couldn't get to grips with the fact that even if you are not counting calories, calories count.

I remember one couple I worked with: the husband was positive he didn't know why he was 5 feet 7 inches tall and weighed in at a whooping 130 kg. I could see the honesty in his face when he told the presenter he was doing everything he could to lose weight. The man had just faced a serious health scare and was begging for help.

The surveillance began. The husband worked for a gas company and travelled around the UK. The secret camera followed him for a week. Every morning, he had a McDonald's – two Sausage and Egg McMuffins with a cappuccino. Mid-morning, he would stop off at a garage and grab a large packet of sweets – Wine Gums, to be exact. Lunch was either fish and chips or a Subway foot-long with a cookie and a large Coke. At dinner, he would have something light, which would be a pub steak and salad, or chicken dinner. This was his routine all week. And the week after.

When the presenter read back to him what he was consuming on a daily basis, he replied, 'I do an active job – I burn up to 3,000 calories on my Fitbit.' She then gave him some numbers. He was over his daily allowance by 500–1,000 calories a day. He was devastated.

This might be an extreme example of why you need to keep an eye on everything you eat, and the trap you can fall into thinking that calories don't count. What you need to understand is that it is easy to grab a bite or a snack here and there and be totally oblivious to how many calories it may contain. This is one of the reasons your weight loss might hit a rocky patch, and becoming more mindful is vital for progress. Think to yourself, 'If Dan had a drone on me, what would he see?'

Be a geek: track steps and standing – every calorie counts

There is a dip in most dads' energy levels at around the same point in the programme. What tends to happen is that they start off carrying at least 20–30 kg more than they should be, so they lose their first 10 kg pretty rapidly.

What happens from this point, if we are not aware of the little gremlins, is that the mind will be in a frenzy, telling you things like, 'If you carry on losing weight like this you'll disappear into thin air.' This is how irrational your mind can be sometimes.

Considering this, when you have experienced some rapid fat loss, part of the reason you might feel it then slows down is because *you* might slow down. The brain has a funny way of doing things; it might sabotage your motivation during your workouts, for example, or reduce your steps throughout the day. The only way you will monitor this is by being rigid with your tracking. Pay close attention to things like your 10,000 steps and how much time you spend sitting. Are you in front of the TV more often than you were? These are the basics we start with, but these are also things we need to maintain to keep going on that fat loss journey.

WHAT'S GOING ON AT WORK?

One dad I worked with had started to become inconsistent with his routine. The tracking system I use with all my clients (Myzone) allows me to see everything, from calories burned to the effort made during every single session. I dropped the guy a message to ask him if everything was OK. I pointed out that the previous month he hadn't missed a session, but that over the past few weeks he had only done four sessions in total. He made every excuse under the sun – and then went on to dismiss them himself, with no prompting from me. He was coming out with things like, 'I just haven't had the time', followed by, 'I know I've got time because I had time last month'.

Eventually (it takes some time with most blokes because we are not supposed to show weakness, right?), he told me that work was stressful, as he was setting up a new company on his own. He said that trying to fit a workout in was adding to his stress.

We discussed a few things and came up with some quick wins that would help him continue with his fat loss. He didn't need to drive to work; it was 20 minutes there and 20 minutes back to cycle.

I revisited the fundamental principle underlying all the systems we use to help with fitness and fat loss: start with one thing. This can also be used to hold on to one thing when the chaos of life creeps in. Sometimes the consistency of just one thing can keep us on track so that when we do have more time, it is easier to go hard and bring the 'A' game back.

Measure, don't weigh

This is probably falling on deaf ears, as the majority of blokes I work with, no matter how many times I tell them, will always measure their fat loss progress by the number on the scales. I have seen so many souls crushed when the number on the scales doesn't even flicker. What are you leaving on the table if you only measure your progress using scales?

Inches. Inches matter. I've known blokes to not lose even a bag of sugar in weight but take 2 inches off their waist. If you have the cash to splash (I know you're a parent, so luxuries like this are few and far between), go to see a professional who can measure fat percentage.

Whatever you do, when it comes to your bodyweight and composition (what your body is made up of – water, tissue, etc), look for progress beyond the scales.

Coaches' corner

It's important to understand that there are a million different factors to consider before we can play the 'I've plateaued' card. I hope all the steps outlined so far have enabled you to grasp the mindset and awareness required to stay on track with your fitness and fat loss pathway. Making continuous adjustments throughout your progress and revaluating what is working and what isn't will keep you 100% in the game. Knowing when your stress levels are elevated because of work or even just life in general is also important. It is too easy to fall back into old habits that you previously used to cope with stress. Remember why you started this in the first place.

Stepping on the scales and feeling disheartened on a weekly basis is enough to send anyone insane, especially when you know you are putting the effort in. Tracking *everything* and being holistic in your measurements will keep your chin up and increase your motivation to stick with it.

STEP 9
Obsessed With Accountability

Many have criticised me in the past for being obsessed and having tunnel vision. Even as a young leading PT in the Royal Navy, those above me in the hierarchy would say I needed to broaden my perspective on fitness. They'd try to send me on various courses that I felt would just distract people from the truth about physical fitness, that you have to earn it.

Through the steps I have presented in this book, I want to demonstrate the fact that there is no substitute for consistency. Being distracted from one thing to focus on another will only lead you further away from achieving serious results.

Becoming obsessed with fitness and taking it seriously can only be a positive thing. I'm sorry to be all clichéd here, but have you heard the saying 'obsessed is what the lazy called dedication'? It's true. Look at every successful person in the world. You won't find a single one who does not obsess about their process, their system. Turn it the other way. At the minute, I'm talking about being obsessed with making your health a priority. What about the people who obsess about the latest Netflix box set? Or worse, those who watch all the British soaps? I mean, come on. How have they got the cheek to say 'You're obsessed with fitness'? Anyway, I'm on my soap box again.

What I have found with the dads I work with is that they become obsessed with accountability. We share all of our workouts together online, each bragging about what we did that day and explaining the obstacles we overcame to get the session done (usually stories about the kids and work). The dads buzz off this and obsess about getting the minimum done daily if they can (minimum being either a 15-minute HIIT (high-intensity interval training) session or a 30-minute power walk). It still surprises me when dads tell me they don't have time to work out and then join the community and seemingly never stop training.

I'M BECOMING OBSESSED. I MIGHT HAVE TO STOP

Here is a story of one of the dads who made the classic error of coming out of the cage too fast and burning out within three weeks. If I'm honest, this happens a lot and is something we have to manage quite often.

His energy in the first week was enough to power the entire south coast. He was like a Duracell bunny on steroids. He came out with statements like, 'Every dad should be doing this,' and, 'I can't believe how much of an impact this is having on my life.' He was hitting it hard, and the other dads were singing his praises and giving him a massive amount of encouragement.

The second week came, and he was still right up there. The other dads were still eagerly awaiting his daily posts and would comment almost instantly when he shared his workout of the day. In the third week, the wind had been taken out of his sails. Throughout the week, the posts became less regular and had less detail. I asked him if there was a problem, and he told me he felt like he was becoming obsessed. I asked him if it was having a negative effect on his life, and he replied that his partner had moaned at him a few times in the evening because when the kids were in bed he was going into the garage to beast a workout.

I asked permission to ask a personal question, and he told me to fire away. I asked, what was his partner doing while he was working out and the kids were in bed? Watching TV, he said. He saw my point. I gave him guidance on how to get his partner onside, and he was off again.

Hull Kingston Rovers vs Hull FC

When the Super You Community first started, the majority of the members were from my home town. (People who know you are more likely to trust you and let you help them.) In my home town, you are either a Hull Kingston

Rovers fan or a Hull FC fan. What does this mean? It means the dads are mad about Rugby League. Not just mad. In some cases, obsessed. There is one dad in the community who insists he will not work with anyone who doesn't support Hull FC (crazy, but true).

Like most dads, they have all played sport at some point and have not filled that fitness void since they hung their boots up. They are still passionate about the sport but don't play anymore. I always get a sense of sadness from them when they talk about the subject.

Every year, if Rovers and FC are in the same league, there is a derby. The teams clash head to head. They go into battle. It's a bloodbath, to say the least, and is regarded as one of the most exciting fixtures of the season. Using Myzone, I looked at how I could make the game even more exciting for the Super You Community by creating a fitness challenge around it.

Within the community, whether or not you were from Hull, you had to choose a side. The result was an almost 50:50 split. The rules were that the team that made the most collective effort would win the competition. How did I measure this? Myzone rewards effort related to heart rate, so the harder you work, the more points you earn by the minute.

The guys went mental for this. Dads were taking days off work. They were motivating each other to work harder. The accountability of not letting the side down was crazy. I saw a different side to what can be achieved when you throw a little healthy competition into the mix.

The Rovers won, by the way. Ever since the competition, when new dads enter the community, they become either Rovers or FC, regardless of where they are from.

Coaches' corner

Obsession is only a negative thing when it becomes detrimental to your health or affects your relationships with others. I've worked with addicts, and I have grown up with addiction in my environment, and let me tell you: when drugs and alcohol are the things you obsess about, that's a problem. There is a difference between being focused on your desired outcome and obsessing to the point where it drives you mad.

Those in your household who are not on the same page as you may give you some resistance and call you out for being 'obsessed'. This is likely just their own insecurities emerging in response to your positive behaviour and your desire to change. Be patient and stick with it.

Accountability to other team members can be a catalyst that ignites a great deal of inspiration to train harder. If you have played a team sport before, think about how you felt towards other team members. Creating that sort of atmosphere in a community is a powerful tool for success in fat loss and fitness.

STEP 10
Sex, Sleep And Rock 'n' Roll

If you haven't seen your penis for a while, the likelihood of you wanting to have sex is probably not at an all-time high. It's the old 'out of sight, out of mind' thing. I've had many messages from dads thanking me because they have got their sex life back on track.

Sex can still sometimes be a taboo subject, but it is a piece in the well-being puzzle. When we feel insecure about out weight and our self-worth is at an all-time low, it can cause all kinds of issues. This is another reason to get lean, get strong and feel awesome.

Another issue that can be a sore subject in a household with little ones is sleep. Sleep deprivation is often the number one factor contributing to arguments in the early days of parenthood. What can you do? If the little tyke is up feeding two or three times a night, there's no compromise – that is just life for that time. That said, I have captured some serious knowledge bombs over the years in terms of how to maximise sleep quality, even if you can't do anything about sleep quantity.

This leads me to the next important piece of the mummy and daddy puzzle. It was almost two years before my partner and I realised that we had not had a single night together without the little one. Those who know us used to call us Bonnie and Clyde back in the day. We were rock 'n' roll, even if I say so myself. After we had our little one, we became more like Thelma and Louise. When we finally did have a night away while nanna took care of things, we exploded (pardon the pun). Having a lie-in in the morning felt alien to us. Our little sausage face would be up two or three times a night right up until she was three years old – nightmare.

GETTING HIS MOJO BACK

A dad approached me about joining the group. He was pretty cut up. He said he felt like his partner was not the slightest bit interested in him and barely touched him these days. I was cut up for him too on reading some of his message, and I did my best to coach him into seeing things from a different perspective. I explained that since he was 120 kg and didn't like what he saw in the mirror, the behaviour he was perceiving in his partner could be a projection of how he felt rather than how his partner felt. He said he'd never looked at it that way before. I explained that when you like what you see in the mirror, you're more likely to smile more often, which will give off a confidence your partner just can't resist.

One morning, about three months after this conversation, I went downstairs at around 5.30am for my usual meditation and worship practice. At 6am, my phone pinged. The dad's name came up in my inbox. I usually wait until around 7.30am to read these sorts of messages, but curiosity got the better of me. The first line read: 'I've just given the missus a knee-trembler in the kitchen. I feel alive!'

I burst out laughing. I was so pleased for the guy. He was over the moon. His weight loss of around 15 kg at this point had made him feel confident in himself once again, and the side effect of this was that he was rampant enough to have sex with his wife in the kitchen before any of the kids got out of bed.

Awesome.

Sleep like a baby? I'm a new parent!

Whoever came up with the saying 'sleep like a baby' needs shooting, and probably never had children. This was a sore subject in our household in the first few years, but especially the first six months. My partner was breastfeeding, and the little one was literally feeding on the hour every hour. It was sending her insane. Although I wasn't involved in the feeding directly, I did my best to support her with cups of tea, chocolate and anything else to help with the stress of being up through the night.

On top of this, at work we kept having in-service training (small workshop-type education things) about how vital it is to get sleep, and its effects on injuries. It was driving me up the wall. And there would always be some celebrity ballbag PT on social media writing that the missing link to fitness is sleep and that if you don't have 8 hours of unbroken sleep per night, you're going to die. (I may be exaggerating a little, but it was enough to piss me off.)

I buried my head in the sand. I stopped following anyone who even mentioned sleep. I was like some sort of keyboard warrior – if I had the time to challenge anyone making fancy posts about sleep, I did. I must have come across as a right bellend.

As time passed and our daughter got older, we started to get a little more sleep. I noticed a massive difference in my mood and my physical activity when I had a good night's rest. At this point, more patients and clients were starting to ask me about sleep. I was a little ignorant on this, so I started to look into it and came across the concept of 'sleep hygiene'. This involved some basic principles around ensuring that even if your quantity of sleep was being affected by something, you took steps to maintain its quality. This has a real positive impact.

There are some simple practices you can put into place that might help, and that most people in the fitness industry agree on:

- Avoid stimulants like caffeine and nicotine too close to bedtime. The effects of caffeine can last for many hours. Nowadays, I have a 3pm cut-off.

- Exercise. This is the obvious quick win for the dads I work with. I often hear that they are sleeping much better after they have been exercising for a few weeks.

- Keep clear of foods that may trigger an unsettled stomach too close to bedtime. You know the types – a vindaloo is probably not the best choice.

- Maintain a regular and relaxing routine (as far as is possible for a parent). Take a warm bath, do some light stretches, maybe do some mindfulness meditation (the Headspace or Calm apps are great). Make sure you hit the sack at the same time most evenings – this is another quick win.

- Control your environment. This plays a huge role. Make sure the lights are low, reduce screen time (you can set a timer in your smartphone settings for this) and switch screens off at least 45 minutes before bed.

After I started paying attention to these basic principles of sleep hygiene, I found that even if my sleep was disturbed, I was still waking up in the morning feeling like I'd had a decent night's sleep.

Rock 'n' roll keeps the fire burning in the soul

House music is something that brought my partner and I closer together. When we first met, we would go hard all weekend in London and go to gigs all over the country. We did some serious raving back in the day (wow, I sound old). We loved music, and not just house music – we went to festivals with rock 'n' roll, indie and all other kinds of tunes. We were close; we were friends and lovers. We had shared interests in almost every aspect of life.

When my partner found out she was pregnant, it was a shock. We weren't expecting it at that stage in our lives, and I certainly wasn't ready to grow up. I could barely look after myself, let alone another human being. When we had our daughter, my partner was faster to step up to the responsibility than I was. I know this because of the frustration she would show towards me in the early months (maybe even years) of the little sausage's life. 'Balls in a vice' comes to mind, and rightly so. For men, it can be difficult at first to understand that life has changed, our partners have changed, and now *we* have to change, too.

Throughout this life transition, fitness was certainly not top of the priority list, but it still had a place in my life. While trying to start a business, hold a job, be a dad, be a son and everything between, I could sense my relationship with my missus had become more about just getting through the day rather than holding hands and attacking the challenges with determination and togetherness. But these are the things that play a huge – if not the most important – role in our mental and physical well-being.

We sat down and discussed the fact that we needed a night or two away, to be the old us. The Bonnie and Clyde who would be up all night raving and chatting about everything and anything – about our dreams and what the future might look like. We finally did get a chance to get away for the night – and my word, did we put the rock into roll. The next week, I noticed that my drive and motivation to train took a different turn. I was excited to get in the gym and be put through my paces.

Keeping the rock 'n' roll in our relationship is a factor affecting our motivation to train, whether we are aware of it or not. When is the last time you took your partner out to wine and dine?

Coaches' corner

Most think fitness is all about lifting weights or running miles. Although these are the mechanical aspects of becoming physically fitter, there is so much more to cultivating the mental resilience to stay consistent with fitness.

Having a comfortable night's sleep and a bedtime routine could be the life hack you need. Even if you have a little one who has you up most of the night, you can at least make sure you maintain the quality of those sacred Zs.

Sex is something that isn't usually discussed with PTs, as it's seen as a private matter. But most clients will happily tell you the ins and outs of all the other excuses for why they might not be motivated, when it could be just as simple as getting their leg over. Losing a bit of timber might just help with this. Keeping the rock 'n' roll in your relationship can affect your motivation – and it's not just about sex, but also some quality 'mummy and daddy time'. I found that getting away for the night with my partner had a huge impact on my training the next week.

Try it.

Review, Take Notes And Get To Work

Like I promised, this is a no-BS approach to fat loss and fitness for dads. I hope I have given you the tools to make fitness a part of your (and your family's) lifestyle. As with any process, it is good practice to go over everything we have been learning throughout the book.

The eleven steps

Step 1: Start with one thing

Every new adventure starts with *one thing*. (I bet you're thinking, this guy and his cliché phrase. What can I say? I'm a cheeseball.)

The prevention of overwhelm in the early phase of the journey is crucial for long-term success. If things get crazy in life and you're not as motivated to get some exercise in the bank, stick to something simple like a power walk or some press-ups. Whatever you choose, just keep moving. You read about how successful Matty has been with this principle, how he started with a daily power walk and ended up completing 28 miles over the Yorkshire Peaks.

Getting started with *one thing* is the aim. Once you have, the rest falls into place.

Step 2: Swap steps for MEPs

Getting into the mindset of becoming a super-geek when it comes to your fitness will only help you on your journey towards your desired results. Recording black and white data on how much you move and how much you eat is going to be a key habit in maximising your fat loss. Within the Super You Community, we use Myzone to gamify fitness and create a supportive and competitive culture that breeds fat loss success. We have had some epic challenges as well as some dads who have taken the bull by the horns, got off their backsides and hit some astonishing achievements – like Frank and Mac. These guys went crazy and still do to this day, to stay on the top page of the monthly Super You challenges.

Step 3: Motion is the lotion

The ability to move is our inheritance, and it is something we must pass on to the next generation. In any new fitness programme, starting with movement is a catalyst for the other factors affecting fitness (nutrition, mindset, etc) to fall into place. Walking more to get clarity and promote mental hygiene is where many of the dads I work with start. Yes, walking burns calories (especially at pace) and slims the waistline, but it also creates head space.

Knowing that every time you move takes a certain degree of effort and therefore burns calories can encourage the mindset of moving more often. Just tidying the house, doing the washing up or getting your hands dirty in the garden all burn calories. Simply being on your feet more often will burn more calories – this is the reason I am an advocate of sit-to-stand desks.

Being mindful of how you spend your time is crucial as a parent, as we tend to have less to manoeuvre with as the nippers get older. That said, just being aware of where you waste time and how you could fit in some exercise can help your waistline.

When you do begin to move on from the one thing you started with, I highly recommend that anyone complete at least one 'leg day' per week. Trust me, this will help with injury prevention, and it burns serious calories. It also helps with increasing your intensity during training, which means torching fat and building muscle.

Step 4: Better mood, better food

Meal plans are not the answer to your fat loss problem. You should understand now that controlling portion size and having knowledge of what foods are calorie-dense will be enough to get you into good habits. Tracking calories does take effort. That said, once you are confident in the amount of food you are consuming and have your calorie intake nailed, it becomes a part of your lifestyle.

Knowing what you have to do to offset the calories you eat is another vital slice of the fitness pie (pun intended). If you are guilty of eating leftovers or overindulging at the weekend, you have to understand what that will cost you in exercise:

Two cans of beer = thirty-minute power walk at a 15- or 13-min/mile pace.

Two chocolate biscuits = 15 minutes of high-intensity training with your heart rate at a minimum of 85%.

Food preparation is not about spending hours slaving in the kitchen on a Sunday. It's about little things like not buying foods you are likely to pick at through the week while watching TV. Or, when you're cooking, putting a little extra in to take to work the next day. Or buying quick meals like supermarket brand microwave rice (always half the price of branded rice) with chopped salad and last night's grilled chicken.

Step 5: Binger vs consistency ninja

The binger vs ninja theme is something I observe with most of my clients. Many set out with the 'start with *one thing*' philosophy in mind. Then, when they have built other things into their lifestyle (doing weights, cycling to work, etc), something might happen at work, or perhaps they go on holiday. Rather than retreating back to the simple thing they started with, they fall into the trap of giving up on everything. They repeat this pattern throughout the year and then wonder why they have made no progress. Or they get distracted by the shakes, pills and other BS in the fitness industry.

Meanwhile, some dads have stuck rigidly to the programme and know that sticking to *one thing* – even when life is chaotic – pays off in the end. These are the dads who get awesome results. Consistency builds momentum, and momentum leads to the unstoppable you.

Step 6: Treat yourself as you would treat your nan

This chapter might have been an uncomfortable read because, as blokes, we tend not to discuss self-respect, our feelings and emotions. This is one of the reasons why suicide rates are higher in males than females. But know this: taking time out and thinking about your breathing might make the difference between walking into the house and losing your shit, or walking into the house and being a calming influence amid the chaos. Knowing when it is time to take yourself away for a bit of fun with the family will also be a key factor in your fat loss.

Step 7: The gremlins of fat loss

Excuses often come down to dads overcomplicating stuff to prevent themselves from starting. They may talk about time as a barrier. When we strip this right back, it's just an overcomplicated excuse.

Running might be the easiest progression from a power walk if the dads want weight loss and it is safe for them to start running (using a programme that builds up from walking). That said, most guys I talk to want the 'lean, like I lift weights' look. Running miles every week isn't going to help achieve this. Power walking along with bodyweight or kettlebell training is something I promote over most programmes, as it allows you to get strong in the comfort of your own home. Bodyweight training or kettlebell training may also solve the problem of an unsupportive partner, as you won't have to spend a couple of hours away from the house training in gyms and all that nonsense.

Being realistic with time frames will save disappointment and set realistic expectations. Be patient and enjoy the process.

Step 8: Plateau is not a place in Greece – nor is it a place in fat loss

Some might criticise my philosophy when it comes to plateaus. But trust me when I say that there is always a stone that has been left unturned. The first, when it comes to fat loss, is forgetting to adjust the calorie tracker to reflect the 10 kg you have lost in the past eight weeks. These sorts of things can really get in the way of fat loss.

It's always awesome to hear about a dad who is the first in the world to defy the law of thermodynamics (burning the calories they put in – or not, apparently). They will tell me that they are doing everything I've told them to and tracking calories like a boss... But they are not counting the two leftover fish fingers, or the caramel macchiato from Starbucks they have first thing in the morning most days. Secret eaters are always the ones who sit at work and tell everyone they have a thyroid problem. They don't.

When it comes to taking the fat loss voyage to the next level, this is the time to really geek out. Being rigid with your step counter is a great start, but if you can get more devices that measure your effort during exercise and give you instant live data, this can step things up a gear in your fat loss and fitness.

Step 9: Obsessed with accountability

As you will have noticed, there are lots of things to consider when seeking to maximise our fat loss and fitness results, and there are some absolutes that cannot be missed. One of these is accountability. Becoming obsessed with accountability and enjoying the fact that effort brings rewards is how things change at speed.

Once they accept that swinging from one programme to another is going to lead to the same disappointment, dads in the Super You Community become obsessed with putting the effort in, turning up and sharing their experiences with the rest of the community. They crave this accountability to one another.

Step 10: Sex, sleep and rock 'n' roll

You might feel like there isn't much more to talk about once you hit the tenth step, but believe me, sex, sleep and rock 'n' roll are important ingredients in the well-being aspect of your fitness and fat loss journey. Having the confidence to take our clothes off in front of our partner, and knowing that our partner finds us attractive, is important to us all, whether we admit it or not.

Getting a good night's kip might be impossible as a parent, but remember the sleep hygiene drills:

- Avoid stimulants like caffeine and nicotine too close to bedtime

- Exercise

- Keep clear of foods that may trigger an unsettled stomach too close to bedtime

- Maintain a regular and relaxing routine (as far as possible for a parent)

- Control your environment

Step 11: Do epic shit to raise money

Imagine going your whole life and barely scratching the surface of what your body is capable of. Most of the dads I come across either tell me they are past it and that their best days are behind them, or they don't believe in themselves full stop. They give no excuses; they just don't feel confident that they can make a positive change to their lives.

In the Super You Community, after we have encouraged the dads to start with *one thing,* they get the wind in their sails. They start believing that the excuses they were making before were just BS – obstacles in their way of becoming the super versions of themselves. Many then challenge themselves further. They start doing epic shit. They start devoting their blood, sweat and tears to a bigger purpose, a cause. They start doing their bit for charities and raising awareness for research projects that can help fight cancer. This is what I call 'next-level shit': where you put yourself in uncomfortable situations, all for a greater cause.

Do Epic Shit To Raise Money

If you never watched Harry Enfield back in the 1990s, then the phrase 'It's for charity, mate' will be wasted on you. (There was a sketch where a radio presenter would take the piss by always doing something for charity.) It is to be admired when someone steps out of their comfort zone to raise awareness and money for a charity. To be frank, it is admirable when someone steps out of their comfort zone to do *anything* worthwhile. What I am talking about here is those who sacrifice time and effort, giving it their all – I don't mean turning your birthday into a freaking charity event on social media.

I have done some epic shit in my life, even if I do say myself. I have put myself in the hurt locker for hours, lost toenails, and literally bled to test where my limits end. That's why, when it comes to charity challenges, it's a win-win situation. You're doing a good thing by raising money, you're getting super-fit, and you have something to focus on.

There is going to come a time where losing fat or building muscle won't have the same effect as it does at the start. Yes, it's important to stay strong and in shape for the activities of daily living, like exploring the outdoors with family, but there will come a time when you will want a challenge, where you will want to put yourself to the test.

Within the Super You Community, there are some amazing dads who have had my jaw dropping with the amount of effort they put into becoming better versions of themselves. Some of them have chosen to do some awesome stuff and make peace with the uncomfortable. There are a few dads that come to mind when I think of this. Here are their inspirational stories.

THE WOLF AND HIS CYCLE AROUND IBIZA

Andy 'The Wolf Man' approached me some time ago. He'd been sitting on the fence, considering whether to join the Super You Community or carry on trying to do everything on his own. He said to me he felt a bit too old and past it. He was 50.

I explained to him that, if anything, it was more important for him to stay fit and in shape than ever. He told me about his worthy goals. One was to run a 10 km race in under 70 minutes for a charity he was an ambassador for. The other was to cycle around the island of Ibiza for the same charity (I nearly invited myself on that one).

For a man who had been nearly 130 kg at one point in his life, this was an epic achievement to aim for. Within the first few months, he went at it like nobody's business, albeit with a few technical difficulties (he is 50, after all). He soon became one of the community's biggest contributors and one of the dads who encouraged everyone else.

He has set goals that are not just about himself. He is constantly sacrificing his time and energy to raise money by devoting blood, sweat and tears to his cause. He is certainly an inspiration to me. He's lost 20 kg, and, more importantly, he is still smashing his fitness goals every single day.

STEP TO IT, MATTY

Matty has come a long way since eating takeaways most evenings and sinking at least sixty cans across the week. In March 2019, he set himself a challenge to hit 10,000 steps a day, every single day of the week. It was for a challenge called 'Walk all Over Cancer', organised by Cancer Research.

During the week, this is easy for Matty, as his job is physically demanding. He would often drop me an inbox of a screenshot of the number of steps he'd completed that day (accountability at its best). That said, come the weekend, getting past 6,000–7,000 steps is difficult for most people. Throw in a few boozy nights, and getting out of the house to do 10,000 steps is the last thing on people's minds.

Matty took on the challenge in style. One weekend, he planned to complete the epic Yorkshire Three Peaks with his friends. That's 28 miles of undulating territory over a period of 8 hours. What can you say to that? Not only did Matty complete thirty-one days consistently; on one of those weekends he walked further than he had ever walked in one go before. After that, I think Matty realised just what he could do if he put his mind to it.

Coaches' corner

We hear stories all the time about heroes who save lives, swim the Atlantic, or cycle across Russia. These are never to be undermined, but it's important to remember that everyone has their own challenges. Everyone has their own limits and hurdles.

My admiration for dads who can manage achievements like those of Matty and The Wolf Man is just as great as it is for the man who can run sixty marathons back to back. Too often, people don't start because they compare their difficulties with those of others. Making such comparisons can help to bring some perspective from time to time, but using them as a reason not to set yourself your own challenges makes for a sad story.

Acknowledgements

I would like to thank all those who have joined me on the journey so far, especially Matthew and Lee.

A big thank you to my wife, Sharlotte, and daughter, Poppy, for their patience during the development of the book.

www.ingramcontent.com/pod-product-compliance
Lightning Source LLC
Chambersburg PA
CBHW031457150726

47990CB00007B/2790